Transforming Emotional Pain and Rediscovering the Self in Anorexia Nervosa

This book presents the SPEAKS approach, an innovative treatment model for anorexia nervosa that primarily combines aspects of Emotion Focused Therapy and Schema Therapy to target struggles with emotion expressed as a "Lost Emotional Self."

An important development for eating disorder treatment models over the last decade is the recognition of difficulties with emotions. This book offers a clear rationale for why emotion is critical in the understanding of anorexia, the blocks to emotional experiencing, as well as how this plays out in regard to the development and experience of anorexia. Structured around five core phases, the treatment framework equips clinicians with practical tools and core therapy tasks designed to help clients reconnect with their emotions. By empowering individuals to articulate their emotional needs, this guide fosters healthier relationships with food and self, ultimately reducing reliance on maladaptive behaviours associated with anorexia.

Transforming Emotional Pain and Rediscovering the Self in Anorexia Nervosa is an essential resource for helping any clinician working in the eating disorder field guide their clients toward emotional healing and self-acceptance.

Dr Anna Oldershaw is a Clinical Psychologist and Reader in Clinical Psychology at the Salomons Institute for Applied Psychology, Canterbury Christ Church University. She has 20 years of clinical and research experience in the field of eating disorders and has published widely in academic journals and books. Anna is an accredited Emotion Focused Therapist, supervisor and international trainer (isEFT), as well as an accredited Schema Therapist (ISST). Anna is Director of the Emotion Focused Therapy Institute of England at Salomons, an isEFT accredited training institute (www.emotionspeaks.co.uk).

Dr Helen Startup is a Consultant Clinical Psychologist with over 20 years of experience working in the field of eating disorders, both as a clinician and as a researcher. She is an accredited CBT therapist (BABCP) and a teacher/trainer of Schema Therapy (ISST), and she co-directs her own schema therapy training school (www.schematherapyschool.co.uk). She has published widely in academic journals and was co-author of the treatment manual for a NICE recommended anorexia nervosa treatment called MANTRA.

Professor Tony Lavender is a Clinical Psychologist with over 40 years of experience working with a range of client groups and a Professor (Emeritus) at Salomons Institute for Applied Psychology, Canterbury Christ Church University. He was the Programme Director for the Clinical Psychology Doctorate at Salomons for 21 years before taking up roles as Dean and Pro-Vice Chancellor (Research). He has published extensively on services and therapies in the areas of psychosis and personality disorder, workforce planning, the history of clinical psychology and more recently anorexia.

'Over half of people with AN do not find treatment that helpful. Addressing cognitions and behaviour in CBT helps some but not all, and a different model is needed. Enter the emotion-focused therapies. SPEAKS is one of these, along with MBT, CFT, ICAT, CAT and FPT. This guidebook provides a really clear and effective guide for potential practitioners. It embodies many elements familiar to experienced therapists: Formulating the problem, motivational enhancement, accessing and resolving trauma or pain and what might be called the butterfly effect, in which the person at last goes forward to a more liberated future. Future RCTs should evaluate therapies such as SPEAKS and broaden the evidence base for treatment of Anorexia Nervosa.'

Prof Paul Robinson, *Consultant Psychiatrist, University College London and Orri Clinic London*

Transforming Emotional Pain and Rediscovering the Self in Anorexia Nervosa

A Clinical Guide

Anna Oldershaw,
Helen Startup, and
Tony Lavender

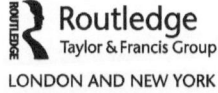
Routledge
Taylor & Francis Group

LONDON AND NEW YORK

Designed cover image: Getty Images @stellalevi

First published 2025
by Routledge
4 Park Square, Milton Park, Abingdon, Oxon OX14 4RN

and by Routledge
605 Third Avenue, New York, NY 10158

Routledge is an imprint of the Taylor & Francis Group, an informa business

British Library Cataloguing-in-Publication Data
A catalogue record for this book is available from the British Library

Library of Congress Cataloging-in-Publication Data
Names: Oldershaw, Anna, author. | Startup, Helen, author. | Lavender, Anthony, author.
Title: Transforming emotional pain and rediscovering the self in anorexia nervosa : a clinical guide / Dr. Anna Oldershaw, Dr. Helen Startup and Professor Tony Lavender.
Description: Abingdon, Oxon ; New York, NY : Routledge, 2025. |
Includes bibliographical references and index.
Identifiers: LCCN 2024052629 (print) | LCCN 2024052630 (ebook) |
ISBN 9781032742434 (hardback) | ISBN 9781032741727 (paperback) |
ISBN 9781003468349 (ebook)
Subjects: LCSH: Anorexia nervosa. | Psychic trauma.
Classification: LCC RC552.A5 O43 2025 (print) | LCC RC552.A5 (ebook) |
DDC 616.85/262–dc23/eng/20250306
LC record available at https://lccn.loc.gov/2024052629
LC ebook record available at https://lccn.loc.gov/2024052630

ISBN: 9781032742434 (hbk)
ISBN: 9781032741727 (pbk)
ISBN: 9781003468349 (ebk)

DOI: 10.4324/9781003468349

Typeset in Times New Roman
by Newgen Publishing UK

Contents

Foreword

This book tells three stories: First it focuses on the story of how the authors developed their innovative model of working with severe anorexia. Second, it tells the story of how therapy for anorexia generally unfolds within the Specialist Psychotherapy with Emotion for Anorexia in Kent and Sussex (SPEAKS) model over five phases. Third, woven throughout the latter chapters, is the charming story of a fictional but representative client, Clara.

The result is honest, bold, practical, earnest and engaging. In this brief foreword, I lay out why you will want to read this book. The authors explain how the SPEAKS model emerged out of a somewhat complicated process combining first the existing quantitative and treatment research literature, emotion research, then two qualitative studies by the SPEAKS team, plus Emotion Focused Therapy (EFT) and Schema Therapy (ST). The result is a treatment that is thoroughly grounded in the literature, informed and guided by qualitative evidence and extensive frontline clinical experience and then channelled through the frameworks of EFT and ST. This integrative origin gives the approach richness and theoretical density; there is nothing superficial or simplistic about it, and it appears to be strongly and deeply grounded in clinical practice.

Throughout, the authors make excellent use of tables to summarise and to provide overviews and alternate ways to process the material. They engage the reader with a vivid, compelling and detailed fictional case study of 'Clara', complete with pre- and post-client drawings.

Another unexpected but welcome feature is the running discussion through the later chapters of the role of neurodivergence in the anorexic population and, more specifically, how to adapt the therapy for different forms of neurodivergent process, including general considerations and relationship formation.

From an EFT perspective, the authors also break new ground not just in describing their approach to anorexic process but also in more general ways, including:

- The description of the specific signs that indicate that the client is moving from one treatment phase to the next.
- A discussion of the structure of different kinds of sessions (active task sessions vs. other sessions), in particular the structure of task sessions.

- The uniquely detailed spelling out for the various therapeutic tasks of what the authors refer to as "Debrief", but which EFT therapists more commonly call *collaborative case formulation work.*
- One of the most interesting and innovative aspects of the authors' presentation is the explicit spelling out of the use of 'two-chair work' repeatedly at different stages of the work, gradually deepening over time, creating a kind of therapeutic spiral, accompanied by detailed specification of differences (and similarities) of the different iterations.
- The clarity and specificity of the stages of the different chair work tasks.

In sum, the authors are to be congratulated for their innovative, down-to-earth description of work with a complex, challenging and important client population. They have listened to their client population, drawn from two key therapeutic approaches and presented the approach in an organised, clinically grounded and illuminating manner.

Professor Robert Elliott
Emeritus Professor of Counselling,
University of Strathclyde (Scotland)
Professor Emeritus of Psychology,
University of Toledo (USA)

Introduction to the SPEAKS Guidebook

This book is the culmination of our clinical experience, research evidence and feedback from those with lived experience of anorexia gathered over more than 20 years. It particularly emerges from our experience of developing and testing an emotion focused intervention for anorexia nervosa since 2016.

The Rationale for an Additional Therapeutic Approach for Anorexia Nervosa

Anorexia nervosa (AN) is a severe mental illness characterised by extreme behaviours of self-starvation, weight loss, and hyperactivity, alongside psychopathology including eating disorder (ED) cognitions such as concerns about eating, weight and shape. It is a one of a group of presentations under the umbrella of EDs, with other difficulties including bulimia nervosa and binge eating disorders. Up to 4% of women will meet Diagnostic & Statistical Manual V (DSM-V) criteria for AN in their lifetime (Galmiche et al., 2019; Smink et al., 2012). AN is associated with poor prognosis and the highest mortality rates of all psychiatric disorders (Demmler et al., 2020). Time spent caregiving for somebody with severe AN is double that for physical health disorders (e.g., cancer) or other mental health disorders (e.g., psychosis; Viana et al., 2013). Thus, substantial clinical, social and economic costs provide a "compelling case for change" in services and treatment (PricewaterhouseCoopers, 2015, p. 9).

First-line treatments for AN are eating disorder focused psychotherapies. These have a core focus on weight restoration, alongside change to ED behaviours and cognitions. For children and adolescents, this is usually a family-based intervention (Fisher et al., 2019). For adults with AN, the National Institute for Health and Care Excellence (NICE; 2017) in the UK recommends specialist psychological 'talking therapy' interventions be considered, including Eating Disorder Focused Cognitive Behavioural Therapy (CBT-ED); Maudsley Anorexia Nervosa Treatment for Adults (MANTRA); Specialist Supportive Clinical Management (SSCM); and Focal Psychodynamic Therapy (FPT).

Emerging evidence suggests that early intervention improves outcomes (Austin et al., 2022). However, individual randomised controlled trials (RCTs) still indicate that there is no superior 'first-line' intervention available, and over 50% of those treated for anorexia remain unwell (Watson & Bulik, 2013). There have been several meta-analyses of treatment for AN over the past two decades which seek to gain a clearer picture on treatment outcomes. These largely conclude that the evidence base for AN treatment is weak and study designs are flawed (Bulik et al., 2007; Hay & Touyz, 2015). Murray and colleagues (2019) examined treatment efficacy for AN in weight and psychological symptoms across 35 RCTs of all treatment types (including psychological and pharmacological), all settings (e.g., inpatient, outpatient), and age groups. They report that, overall, there was a significant effect of treatment (including specialist ED treatment) on weight outcomes at end of treatment, but no significant change in psychological symptom outcomes. At follow-up, there was no effect of treatment on weight or psychological outcomes.

Meanwhile, Zeeck et al. (2018) attempted to clarify findings by completing a meta-analysis of 18 RCTs focusing on weight change following individual psychotherapeutic interventions specifically across settings and age groups. The results indicate that, for adults with AN, no specific ED specialist psychotherapeutic intervention resulted in significantly better weight gain outcomes as compared with a control comparator of clinical management (SSCM). They did not examine psychological outcomes. The finding is expanded by van den Berg and colleagues (2019), whose meta-analysis of 15 studies found that specialist psychological treatments show no advantage over control comparisons on measures of weight gain, ED psychopathology or quality of life.

Most recently, Solmi and colleagues (2021) conducted a network analysis on 16 RCTs to compare change following psychological interventions for adults with anorexia. The reviewed outcomes including body mass index (BMI), ED symptoms and all-cause dropout rate. The review found that no intervention outperformed treatment as usual for either weight (measured by BMI) or ED psychopathology, although dropout rate was lowest for CBT.

Adding to concerns over the evidence base is the fact that prognosis and outcomes from treatment appear further impeded for people with significant comorbidity or longer illness duration (Hambleton et al., 2022; Meule et al., 2023). At least 60% of those struggling with an ED have significant personality disorder traits (e.g., emotional dysregulation, significant relational struggles) and many have anxiety, depression, OCD and other Axis 1 presentations (Link et al., 2017; Miller et al., 2021). Up to 40% of people with AN are autistic (and many more may be otherwise neurodivergent) which can complicate their presentation or intervention needs (Nimbley et al., 2023). Furthermore, it is known that treatments of standard length (20–30 sessions) are less effective for those with longer illness durations (Ambwani et al., 2020; Schmidt et al., 2015). These difficulties in meeting need for people with AN have only been exacerbated by the Covid-19 pandemic, which has seen a rise in incidence rates, level of symptomatology and hospital admissions (Gilsbach et al., 2022; Katzman, 2021; Vyver et al., 2023).

In summary, our ability to treat adults with AN remains limited despite persistent efforts and developments in this and other fields of psychotherapy, all while in the face of increasing demand for AN treatments. This lack of effective treatments is a significant concern, particularly for those who don't respond to standard treatments (Treasure et al., 2021). As such, AN is notoriously considered 'difficult to treat', and there is an enduring urgent need to develop innovative and engaging interventions (Bulik, 2014; Solmi et al., 2021) while targeting unique development and maintenance factors (Kass et al., 2013). In particular, a gap remains in the existing evidence base for an effective therapeutic intervention for those with comorbidities and longer illness durations, sometimes referred to as those with 'severe and enduring' illness.

The Rationale for Focusing on Emotion in Therapy for AN

Emotional experience as a factor in the development and maintenance of AN has been recognised from its earliest descriptions in medical literature. In 1871, a patient with AN was reported to *"suffer from some emotions she avows or conceals"* (Charles Lasègue cited in Vandereycken & Van Deth, 1990). A century later, women with AN were described as having underlying deficiencies in the identification of emotional states and responses (Bruch, 1962). A link between avoiding or controlling emotional experience and the behavioural expression of AN is clear. Potential emotion is avoided by eliciting predictable and controllable behavioural patterns from others (Treasure et al., 2016); cognitive distraction from negative thoughts/emotion is achieved though focus on food, eating, weight, shape, exercise and purging behaviours, as well as via cognitive processes such as worry and rumination (Startup et al., 2013; Sternheim et al., 2015). AN (at least initially) appears to meet psychological and emotional needs by affording a sense of achievement thereby reducing distress (Gulliksen et al., 2017). In the starvation state, suppressed physiological experience is valued for its numbing effect on emotion (Miller et al., 2009; Miller et al., 2003; Serpell et al., 2004), while starvation and emaciation enable a non-verbal expression of distress (Serpell et al., 2004). Working with emotion is highlighted as a promising target area for therapies (Sala et al., 2016) and is increasingly incorporated into developments of psychotherapy interventions for adults with AN (Dolhanty & Greenberg, 2009; Hibbs et al., 2021; Schmidt & Treasure, 2014; Tchanturia et al., 2015; Wildes & Marcus, 2011). However, the impact of working with emotion on therapeutic outcomes remains unclear, and it is uncertain to what extent emotional difficulties are successfully targeted by these interventions.

The SPEAKS Approach

The complexity of AN and the inherent risk in this presentation can impede the focus and progression of psychological therapy as therapists attend to many competing factors and symptoms. Intervention development and application difficulties in mental health more broadly are argued to reflect an 'everything is relevant' approach, meaning all possible factors are sought to be resolved, which results in a lack of clarity and efficiency in achieving desired change and, consequently, often not effectively targeting identified variables (Kendler & Campbell, 2009). This lack of focus upon how best to target identified variables is associated with an absence of 'mechanistic' understandings of change in AN, argued to have undermined previous development of evidence-based interventions for this client group (Kaye & Bulik, 2021). Treatments of other complex disorders have improved outcomes by focusing on a clearly defined model with key putative maintaining process, hypothesised to subsequently impact symptomatology (c.f. targeting worry to effect change across psychosis symptoms; Freeman et al., 2015).

Our proposal in beginning to develop a new intervention was that reducing complexity of therapeutic foci is crucial when working with AN, particularly for those with established and enduring AN. Furthermore, improved understanding of the possible mechanisms of change in treatment and elucidating clear hypothesised change processes would be crucial. The Specialist Psychotherapy with Emotion for Anorexia in Kent and Sussex (SPEAKS) programme thus designed an 'interventionist-causal model approach' (Kendler & Campbell, 2009) by focusing on a core clearly defined model targeting one key putative maintaining process – namely experience of emotion and emotional vulnerability – in order to improve presenting symptomatology. We sought to understand psychotherapeutic targets and mechanisms of change from the "bottom-up", learning from lived experiences of change and its facilitation, thus integrating a 'persons-based' approach (Yardley, Ainsworth et al., 2015; Yardley, Morrison et al., 2015). Ultimately, we worked towards developing an emotion-focused intervention for adults with anorexia (SPEAKS intervention) and then tested it in a feasibility trial. Our goals were to create an evidence-based, acceptable, and feasible emotion-focused psychotherapeutic intervention for adults with AN with a-priori testable change process hypotheses.

Overview of This Book

In this book, we detail the development of the SPEAKS intervention for anorexia and associated research, before providing an in-depth description of its application to support therapists in delivering the approach in practice.

Section I of this book is dedicated to outlining the theoretical underpinning and preliminary research evidence in support of the SPEAKS approach. Chapter 1 describes the background evidence, including research we conducted to better understand the emotion change processes associated with recovery from AN. We introduce our theory that many risk and maintenance factors for AN reflect an underpinning explanation of emotional processing difficulties which lead to a lost sense of 'emotional self', and once established, AN becomes 'self-perpetuating', with this 'lost sense of emotional self' relentlessly deepening.

In Chapter 2, we present a detailed description of the underlying theory of EFT and ST, including key concepts of relevance to the SPEAKS approach. We draw together our SPEAKS development work with the theory and practice of EFT and ST to outline the SPEAKS emotion focused conceptualisation and our hypothesised change processes. We explain how this approach focuses on working with, but moving past, the symptom-level presentation to target underlying emotional vulnerability, namely core pain and associated unmet need, and facilitate emotion processing and transformation. Therefore, in this chapter, we present our model of change in SPEAKS therapy.

Chapter 3 goes on to describe the SPEAKS research evidence gathered to date, including both findings from a multi-site single arm feasibility trial and integrated research designs testing our change process hypotheses.

Section II of this book presents a therapist manual for SPEAKS delivery. We describe this as a guidebook in recognition of the fact that it is to be used in a flexible way, with responsiveness to experiential markers and emerging needs of clients, while also offering a guided outline for the overall process of therapy. For a clinician delivering SPEAKS, having a core therapeutic training is essential and having specific training in an experiential and relational therapy is recommended.

Chapter 4 explains the five phases of SPEAKS, the goals of each phase and when moving to work within the next phase is indicated. It discusses the structure of a typical therapy session within the context of an experiential approach to therapy.

A detailed description of SPEAKS therapy begins in Chapter 5 by outlining SPEAKS Phase 1: Formulation and Engagement. This phase establishes the groundwork for therapy with key consideration given to building a warm, safe therapeutic relationship central to facilitating change and developing the case formulation using a "mode map" approach which anchors subsequent treatment. In Chapter 6, we discuss how we seek to work to stabilise symptoms but ultimately move past these during Phase 2: Seeing through and Moving past the Façade. Here we offer ways to support clients to enhance motivation for change and reduce a sense of 'stuckness', leading to increased trust in and engagement with the therapy process. Throughout each phase we use the case example of 'Clara' to bring to life the clinical description and to support the reader to have a practical, relational, and felt sense of the SPEAKS therapeutic journey.

Chapter 7 focuses on Phase 3: Connecting with Core Pain, with emphasis on how to support clients to begin to do this using containing and safe approaches. Chapter 8 goes on to describe the process of transforming painful experiences during Phase 4: Resolving Core Pain.

Phases 3 and 4 embody the core emotional change processes inherent in the intervention. Following these phases, the hope is that clients are now beginning to connect their transformed emotional experience to alternative intra- and interpersonal ways of responding which reflect a more resilient and integrated sense of self – the healthy Adult – now acting to get needs met in healthy ways. In chapter 9, we discuss ways to consolidate this newly emerging sense of self and its self-agency and self-efficacy to develop the client's new experiences within the world and relationships during the final phase of SPEAKS, Phase 5: The Emergence of the 'Real Me'.

References

Ambwani, S., Cardi, V., Albano, G., Cao, L., Crosby, R. D., Macdonald, P., Schmidt, U., & Treasure, J. (2020). A multicenter audit of outpatient care for adult anorexia nervosa: Symptom trajectory, service use, and evidence in support of "early stage" versus "severe and enduring" classification. *International Journal of Eating Disorders, 53*(8), 1337–1348.

Austin, A., Flynn, M., Shearer, J., Long, M., Allen, K., Mountford, V. A., Glennon, D., Grant, N., Brown, A., & Franklin-Smith, M. (2022). The first episode rapid early intervention for eating disorders-upscaled study: clinical outcomes. *Early Intervention in Psychiatry, 16*(1), 97–105.

Bruch, H. (1962). Perceptual and conceptual disturbances in anorexia nervosa. *Psychosomatic Medicine, 24*(2), 187–194.

Bulik, C. M. (2014). The challenges of treating anorexia nervosa. *The Lancet, 383*(9912), 105–106.

Bulik, C. M., Berkman, N. D., Brownley, K. A., Sedway, J. A., & Lohr, K. N. (2007). Anorexia nervosa treatment: a systematic review of randomized controlled trials. *International Journal of Eating Disorders, 40*(4), 310–320.

Demmler, J. C., Brophy, S. T., Marchant, A., John, A., & Tan, J. O. (2020). Shining the light on eating disorders, incidence, prognosis and profiling of patients in primary and secondary care: national data linkage study. *The British Journal of Psychiatry, 216*(2), 105–112.

Dolhanty, J., & Greenberg, L. S. (2009). Emotion-focused therapy in a case of anorexia nervosa. *Clinical Psychology & Psychotherapy: An International Journal of Theory & Practice, 16*(4), 336–382.

Fisher, C. A., Skocic, S., Rutherford, K. A., & Hetrick, S. E. (2019). Family therapy approaches for anorexia nervosa. *Cochrane Database of Systematic Reviews* (5).

Freeman, D., Dunn, G., Startup, H., Pugh, K., Cordwell, J., Mander, H., Černis, E., Wingham, G., Shirvell, K., & Kingdon, D. (2015). Effects of cognitive behaviour therapy for worry on persecutory delusions in patients with psychosis (WIT): A parallel, single-blind, randomised controlled trial with a mediation analysis. *The Lancet Psychiatry, 2*(4), 305–313.

Galmiche, M., Déchelotte, P., Lambert, G., & Tavolacci, M. P. (2019). Prevalence of eating disorders over the 2000–2018 period: A systematic literature review. *The American Journal of Clinical Nutrition, 109*(5), 1402–1413.

Gilsbach, S., Plana, M. T., Castro-Fornieles, J., Gatta, M., Karlsson, G. P., Flamarique, I., Raynaud, J.-P., Riva, A., Solberg, A.-L., & van Elburg, A. A. (2022). Increase in admission rates and symptom severity of childhood and adolescent anorexia nervosa in Europe during the COVID-19 pandemic: Data from specialized eating disorder units in different European countries. *Child and Adolescent Psychiatry and Mental Health, 16*(1), 46.

Gulliksen, K. S., Nordbø, R. H., Espeset, E. M., Skårderud, F., & Holte, A. (2017). Four pathways to anorexia nervosa: Patients' perspective on the emergence of AN. *Clinical Psychology & Psychotherapy, 24*(4), 846–858.

Hambleton, A., Pepin, G., Le, A., Maloney, D., Touyz, S., & Maguire, S. (2022). Psychiatric and medical comorbidities of eating disorders: Findings from a rapid review of the literature. *Journal of Eating Disorders*, *10*(1), 132.

Hay, P., & Touyz, S. (2015). Treatment of patients with severe and enduring eating disorders. *Current Opinion in Psychiatry*, *28*(6), 473–477.

Hibbs, R., Pugh, M., & Fox, J. R. (2021). Applying emotion-focused therapy to work with the "anorexic voice" within anorexia nervosa: A brief intervention. *Journal of Psychotherapy Integration*, *31*(4), 327–347.

Kass, A. E., Kolko, R. P., & Wilfley, D. E. (2013). Psychological treatments for eating disorders. *Current Opinion in Psychiatry*, *26*(6), 549–555.

Katzman, D. K. (2021). The COVID-19 pandemic and eating disorders: A wake-up call for the future of eating disorders among adolescents and young adults. *Journal of Adolescent Health*, *69*(4), 535–537.

Kaye, W. H., & Bulik, C. M. (2021). Treatment of patients with anorexia nervosa in the US—A crisis in care. *JAMA Psychiatry*, *78*(6), 591–592.

Kendler, K. S., & Campbell, J. (2009). Interventionist causal models in psychiatry: Repositioning the mind–body problem. *Psychological Medicine*, *39*(6), 881–887.

Link, T. M., Beermann, U., Mestel, R., & Gander, M. (2017). Treatment outcome in female in-patients with anorexia nervosa and comorbid personality disorders prevalence-therapy drop out and weight gain. *Psychotherapie, Psychosomatik, medizinische Psychologie*, *67*(9–10), 420–430.

Meule, A., Kolar, D. R., Rauh, E., & Voderholzer, U. (2023). Comparing illness duration and age as predictors of treatment outcome in female inpatients with anorexia nervosa. *Eating Disorders*, *31*(3), 274–284.

Miller, A. E., Racine, S. E., & Klonsky, E. D. (2021). Symptoms of anorexia nervosa and bulimia nervosa have differential relationships to borderline personality disorder symptoms. *Eating Disorders*, *29*(2), 161–174.

Miller, S. P., Erickson, S. J., Branom, C., & Steiner, H. (2009). Habitual response to stress in recovering adolescent anorexic patients. *Child Psychiatry and Human Development*, *40*, 43–54.

Miller, S. P., Redlich, A. D., & Steiner, H. (2003). The stress response in anorexia nervosa. *Child Psychiatry and Human Development*, *33*, 295–306.

Murray, S. B., Quintana, D. S., Loeb, K. L., Griffiths, S., & Le Grange, D. (2019). Treatment outcomes for anorexia nervosa: A systematic review and meta-analysis of randomized controlled trials. *Psychological Medicine*, *49*(4), 535–544.

National Institute for Health and Care Excellence (2017). *Eating Disorders: Recognition and Treatment*. (NICE Guidelines NG69). https://www.nice.org.uk/guidance/ng69

Nimbley, E., Gillespie-Smith, K., Duffy, F., Maloney, E., Ballantyne, C., & Sharpe, H. (2023). "It's not about wanting to be thin or look small, it's about the way it feels": an IPA analysis of social and sensory differences in autistic and non-autistic individuals with anorexia and their parents. *Journal of Eating Disorders*, *11*(1), 89.

PricewaterhouseCoopers. (2015). *The costs of eating disorders: social health and economic impacts*. https://www.b-eat.co.uk/assets/000/000/302/The_costs_of_eating_disorders_Final_original.pdf.

Sala, M., Heard, A., & Black, E. A. (2016). Emotion-focused treatments for anorexia nervosa: A systematic review of the literature. *Eating and Weight Disorders-Studies on Anorexia, Bulimia and Obesity*, *21*, 147–164.

Schmidt, U., Magill, N., Renwick, B., Keyes, A., Kenyon, M., Dejong, H., Lose, A., Broadbent, H., Loomes, R., & Yasin, H. (2015). The Maudsley Outpatient Study of Treatments for Anorexia Nervosa and Related Conditions (MOSAIC): Comparison of the Maudsley Model of Anorexia Nervosa Treatment for Adults (MANTRA) with specialist supportive clinical management (SSCM) in outpatients with broadly defined anorexia nervosa: A randomized controlled trial. *Journal of Consulting and Clinical Psychology*, *83*(4), 796–807.

Schmidt, U., & Treasure, J. (2014). The Maudsley Model of Anorexia Nervosa Treatment for Adults (MANTRA): Development, key features, and preliminary evidence. *Journal of Cognitive Psychotherapy*, *28*(1), 48–71.

Serpell, L., Teasdale, J. D., Troop, N. A., & Treasure, J. (2004). The development of the P-CAN, a measure to operationalize the pros and cons of anorexia nervosa. *International Journal of Eating Disorders*, *36*(4), 416–433.

Smink, F. R., Van Hoeken, D., & Hoek, H. W. (2012). Epidemiology of eating disorders: incidence, prevalence and mortality rates. *Current Psychiatry Reports*, *14*(4), 406–414.

Solmi, M., Wade, T., Byrne, S., Del Giovane, C., Fairburn, C., Ostinelli, E., De Crescenzo, F., Johnson, C., Schmidt, U., & Treasure, J. (2021). Comparative efficacy and acceptability of psychological interventions for the treatment of adult outpatients with anorexia nervosa: A systematic review and network meta-analysis. *The Lancet Psychiatry*, *8*(3), 215–224.

Startup, H., Lavender, A., Oldershaw, A., Stott, R., Tchanturia, K., Treasure, J., & Schmidt, U. (2013). Worry and rumination in anorexia nervosa. *Behavioural and Cognitive Psychotherapy*, *41*(3), 301–316.

Sternheim, L., Startup, H., & Schmidt, U. (2015). Anxiety-related processes in anorexia nervosa and their relation to eating disorder pathology, depression and anxiety. *Advances in Eating Disorders: Theory, Research and Practice*, *3*(1), 13–19.

Tchanturia, K., Doris, E., Mountford, V., & Fleming, C. (2015). Cognitive Remediation and Emotion Skills Training (CREST) for anorexia nervosa in individual format: self-reported outcomes. *BMC Psychiatry*, *15*, 1–6.

Treasure, J., Oyeleye, O., Bonin, E. M., Zipfel, S., & Fernandez-Aranda, F. (2021). Optimising care pathways for adult anorexia nervosa. What is the evidence to guide the provision of high-quality, cost-effective services? *European Eating Disorders Review*, *29*(3), 306–315.

Treasure, J., Smith, G., & Crane, A. (2016). *Skills-based caring for a loved one with an eating disorder: The new Maudsley method*. Routledge.

van den Berg, E., Houtzager, L., de Vos, J., Daemen, I., Katsaragaki, G., Karyotaki, E., Cuijpers, P., & Dekker, J. (2019). Meta-analysis on the efficacy of psychological treatments for anorexia nervosa. *European Eating Disorders Review*, *27*(4), 331–351.

Vandereycken, W., & Van Deth, R. (1990). A tribute to Lasègue's description of anorexia nervosa (1873), with completion of its English translation. *The British Journal of Psychiatry*, *157*(6), 902–908.

Viana, M. C., Gruber, M. J., Shahly, V., Alhamzawi, A., Alonso, J., Andrade, L. H., ... & Kessler, R. C. (2013). Family burden related to mental and physical disorders in the world: Results from the WHO World Mental Health (WMH) surveys. *Revista brasileira de psiquiatria*, *35*(2), 115–125.

Vyver, E., Han, A. X., Dimitropoulos, G., Patten, S. B., Devoe, D. J., Marcoux-Louie, G., & Katzman, D. K. (2023). The COVID-19 pandemic and Canadian pediatric tertiary care hospitalizations for anorexia nervosa. *Journal of Adolescent Health, 72*(3), 344–351.

Watson, H., & Bulik, C. (2013). Update on the treatment of anorexia nervosa: Review of clinical trials, practice guidelines and emerging interventions. *Psychological Medicine, 43*(12), 2477–2500.

Wildes, J. E., & Marcus, M. D. (2011). Development of emotion acceptance behavior therapy for anorexia nervosa: A case series. *International Journal of Eating Disorders, 44*(5), 421–427.

Yardley, L., Ainsworth, B., Arden-Close, E., & Muller, I. (2015). The person-based approach to enhancing the acceptability and feasibility of interventions. *Pilot and Feasibility Studies, 1*(1), 1–7.

Yardley, L., Morrison, L., Bradbury, K., & Muller, I. (2015). The person-based approach to intervention development: application to digital health-related behavior change interventions. *Journal of Medical Internet Research, 17*(1), e4055.

Zeeck, A., Herpertz-Dahlmann, B., Friederich, H.-C., Brockmeyer, T., Resmark, G., Hagenah, U., Ehrlich, S., Cuntz, U., Zipfel, S., & Hartmann, A. (2018). Psychotherapeutic treatment for anorexia nervosa: A systematic review and network meta-analysis. *Frontiers in Psychiatry, 9*, 158.

Section 1

Chapter 1

Anorexia and a
'Lost Emotional Self'

Understanding the Emotions 'Problem'

To develop the Specialist Psychotherapy with Emotion for Anorexia in Kent and Sussex (SPEAKS) theoretical model of change and subsequent therapeutic intervention, the SPEAKS research programme began by seeking an understanding of the 'problem' with regards to emotional difficulties experienced by people with anorexia nervosa (AN). Evidence highlighted through previously published systematic reviews of empirical data regarding emotional difficulties and AN (Lavender et al., 2015; Oldershaw et al., 2011; Oldershaw et al., 2015) was synthesised with published qualitative data, as well as broader evolutionary and clinical theories of emotions. This synthesis indicated that, relative to unaffected people, people with AN experience emotional awareness difficulties, including reduced emotional clarity and difficulty naming emotions (alexithymia), as well as high levels of shame and self-disgust. Meta-level processes also revealed high levels of negative beliefs about having or expressing emotion, alongside beliefs about personal defectiveness, incompetence, and coping styles including social isolation and suppressing one's own emotions and needs to please others (Oldershaw et al., 2015).

Findings support the notion that emotional avoidance and unhelpful over-regulation strategies play a central role in AN and predict clinical outcomes following treatment (Oldershaw et al., 2018). This includes coping strategies connected to eating disorder behaviours (Arcelus et al., 2013; Brockmeyer et al., 2014; Dolhanty & Greenberg, 2009; Schmidt & Treasure, 2014; Wildes & Marcus, 2011). Common emotion regulation methods employed include avoidance of emotion triggers by avoiding or modifying social interaction (e.g. using submissiveness or self-subjugation); worry and rumination processes, and the suppression of emotion. People with AN are also disproportionately reliant upon the feedback of others for reassurance and emotion regulation (e.g., via social comparison) (Oldershaw et al., 2015). As such, these findings point to a maintenance model of AN as underpinned by difficulties with emotional experience promoting emotional avoidance and over-regulation (Oldershaw et al., 2015). Furthermore it is suggested that these strategies emerge from early life and/or developmental factors and resultant schemata that leave the person vulnerable to experiencing emotion as overwhelming

DOI: 10.4324/9781003468349-2

and confusing. Emotion regulation strategies, including eating disorder (ED) behaviours, develop as a means to control and prevent triggering (feared) emotion. Strategies developed are perceived as useful in the first instance, generating an initial emotion decrease. Ultimately, however, they are maladaptive methods of controlling and regulating emotion serving only to trigger further negative emotional experience and reinforce negative beliefs and schemata, thereby increasing reliance upon (maladaptive) emotion regulation strategies: hence a vicious cycle develops and is maintained (Oldershaw et al., 2015).

Emotions as Fundamental to our Sense of Self

Emotions are fundamental to our human experience and are understood as learnt or instinctive responses to external or internal stimuli informing about our immediate environments, relationships, and crucially, our needs. They rapidly alert us to significant current and emerging information in an environment or relationship, preparing us for action in order to meet our associated needs; this enables us to survive and thrive. We are born with the capacity to be angry, sad, and afraid. The capacity to experience those emotions is significantly affected by our experience of others, particularly caregivers, reactions to those emotions, and our own internal (conscious and unconscious) and external responses. These reactions and responses to emotions become an integral part of our existence and the basis for our sense of self (Damasio, 2003). Difficulties with emotion can thus become so pervasive and damaging that they undermine our sense of self (Damasio, 2003).

Our emotional experience emerges out of physical arousal, including interoceptive and proprioceptive experiences, alongside processes such as neural activation (Barrett et al., 2007) and emotional memory networks (Greenberg, 2004). Interoceptive emotion signals afford us a mental representation of selfhood experienced within the body – 'a material me' (Seth, 2013). Thus identity is rooted in one's connection with the body with emotion being fundamental to that construction and organisation of an autonomously directed 'self' via a process of nonconscious emotional experience (Hatch et al., 2010). However, when we cannot access emotional experience grounded in our bodies ('a material me'), we lose our sense of self. People with AN lack interoceptive perception of their own body and the internal bodily sensations which give rise to the basic form of self-awareness and emotion perception (Gaudio et al., 2014; Stanghellini et al., 2018). There is consequently a lack of confidence in the body as a trustworthy source of information via interoceptive awareness (Monteleone et al., 2021). Of note, neurodivergent people (who are very overrepresented in eating disorder populations; Huke et al., 2013) experience a range of sensory differences which may exacerbate such difficulties, including poor integration of interoceptive information (Loureiro et al., 2024).

We suggest that AN emerges in this context of vague and overwhelming emotional experience, both to regulate emotion (Oldershaw et al., 2015) and to regain a sense of bodily self, focusing on tangible markers of identity (body, weight, and shape) (Oldershaw et al., 2019), defined by the other's gaze and external appearance (Monteleone et al., 2017). As such, AN has been referred to as a 'false self' (Bruch, 1982), arising due to an otherwise unstable and fragile self (Karwautz et al., 2001) unable to integrate bodily experience (Amianto et al., 2016). This aligns with findings that significant disturbance in identity is a central maintenance factor for AN and resolution of such difficulties is crucial for recovery (Croce et al., 2024). These data informed and culminated in our proposal that many risk and maintenance factors for AN may be unified by an underpinning explanation of emotional processing difficulties ultimately leading to a 'lost sense of emotional self'., that is, a person struggling to navigate the world, themselves and others, without an emotional conductor to guide them through life's symphony, instead becoming increasingly reliant upon the feedback of others (the 'audience'). We hypothesised that the emergence and integration of an 'emotional self' which can flexibly and adaptively listen to and direct an individual's needs and relationships could be a primary goal of therapy for adults with established AN (Oldershaw et al., 2019).

SPEAKS Model Development Work

This initial theory work culminated in the identification of a clear goal for SPEAKS therapy: regaining a sense of emotional self, integrated within the body. Furthermore, it illuminated gaps in the evidence about the process of emotional change linked to recovery from anorexia. Evidence highlighted emotional and social difficulties for (a) those currently ill and (b) what had improved once recovered; however, evidence for the change process in getting from (a) to (b) was lacking. In order to better understand how to facilitate change, and support clients to reconnect with their 'emotional self', our next steps focused on researching emotional change processes associated with AN recovery. We firstly considered *what* needed to change and in what order, and then what processes might best facilitate such change (*how*).

The 'What' of Emotional Change Processes Linked to Recovery

To gain insight into the processes of emotional change, semi-structured interviews with nine adult women in different stages of recovery from AN were conducted by an independent researcher blind to the 'lost self' hypothesis to reduce influencing data interpretation. Constructivist grounded theory analysis developed a theory of emotional change (Figure 1). Ten major categories emerged, clustered into three super categories, reflecting distinct but interrelated phases of participants' journeys toward recovery: (1) *Coping in a world of uncertainty* (perceiving emotions negatively and using ways of coping, including AN, to

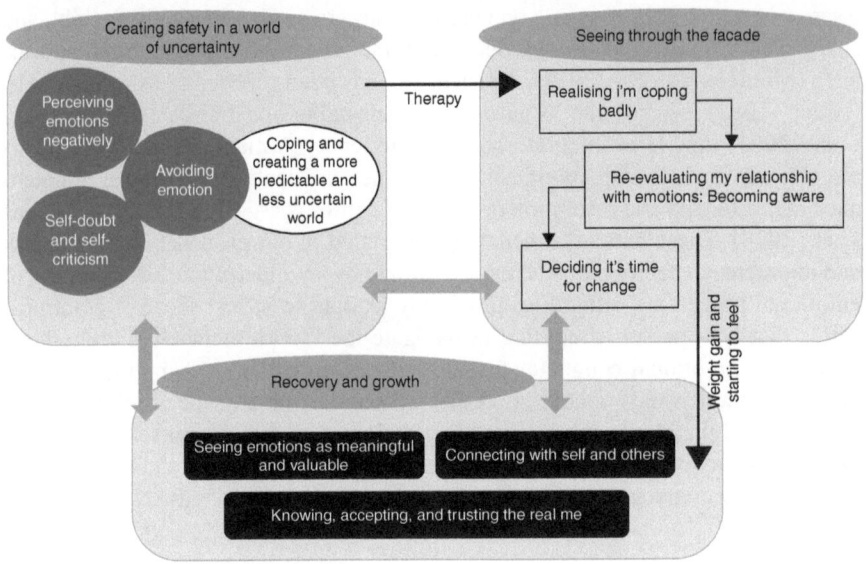

Figure 1.1 The process of emotional change associated with recovery, reproduced with permission from Drinkwater et al. (2022).

avoid emotion and create predictability), (2) *Seeing through the façade of anorexia* (the realisation that, while drawing on strategies to cope, avoid, block, distract from, or displace emotions had felt helpful before, this had limits), and (3) *Recovery and growth* (seeing emotions as important and valuable; connecting self–self and self–others; knowing, liking, and accepting the 'Real Me') (Drinkwater et al., 2022).

This work highlighted a process of change starting with gaining meta-perspective on current ways of coping – moving from a position of *creating safety* to *seeing through the façade of anorexia*. This facilitated the beginning of a new motivation for finding different ways to manage in life. Through engagement with therapy, people developed a new relationship with emotions where they were now seen as meaningful and valuable, rather than something feared and avoided. Here was the emergence of an authentic self that could leave the ED behind (*recovery and growth*). These findings support the notion that emotional change is of relevance to recovery from AN and highlight the pursuit of an authentic connection with self and identity (finding *the 'Real Me'*). The concept of developing the 'Real Me' connected to core emotion and underpinning needs paralleled our proposed 'lost sense of emotional self' theory whilst outlining a clearer sense of important steps to reach that goal. This aligned with research from those with lived experience who described recovery as being dependent upon development of insight into the ED and acceptance of the self, as well as contingent upon finding meaning and purpose, empowerment and self-compassion (Bardone-Cone et al., 2018; Bardone-Cone et al., 2020; Stockford et al., 2019).

The 'How' of Emotional Change Processes Linked to Recovery

To further understand how to best approach and facilitate identified emotional change processes, we sought lived experiences of (i) people with a history of AN, (ii) family members of people with lived experience, and (iii) professionals working psychotherapeutically with people with AN (Davies et al., in prep). Focus groups and qualitative interviews utilised purposive samples recruited via NHS services and from advertisements within local networks of eating disorder support groups. Twenty-eight participants, comprising twelve people with anorexia, seven carers and nine therapists, engaged in focus groups or individual interviews. A thematic analysis following Braun and Clarke's six step process (Braun & Clarke, 2012) generated themes of *key emotions experienced, how emotional change happens, and the therapeutic stance.*

Key emotions of *anxiety*, *guilt*, *shame*, and *abandonment* (being left alone with emotion) were indicated as prevalent and recognised as important foci for therapy, which aligns with other reports of these being prevalent persistent emotions experienced by people with AN (Oldershaw et al., 2015).

Accepting and validating emotion was described as a channel for change,

It's okay to have your own emotion and feel. (client participant)

… what I felt … it wasn't bad, you know, it was valid. (client participant)

If you are speaking to the emotion, you have a conversation at all times, and that is very, very helpful, because that word again, it shows compassion and it shows respect, and just that understanding. (carer participant)

This occurred alongside removing of blocks to support clients to acknowledge, identify and express difficult feelings.

I blocked feelings and emotions for so long and when I learned to start acknowledging them and identifying them, well, it gave me a little bit of a platform to start working on, and it gave me, like, a starting point. (client participant)

So when I came to feel more free in saying when I'm angry, because I was so used to being quiet and submissive and just trying to like disappear from everyone's life than my own … to have a kind of presence to actually say what I feel has been a real battle. Erm and until I could address that, yeah, I couldn't even think about food. (client participant)

Participants described the need for a therapy that focused on emotions to **go beyond finding strategies for emotion regulation and instead to promote emotions as meaningful and seek to understand underlying reasons and needs.**

I don't identify necessarily with regulating emotion. It could be a response to, you know, feeling overwhelmed or feeling out of control, or feeling broken. (client participant)

Participants thus highlighted the value of using therapy to **explore feelings, where they came from, what they meant, and using that to guide** a better understanding of the self.

> *Being able to understand the root emotions and then how they can change over, even not over that long, but so that you can kind of understand yourself a bit more.* (client participant)

The therapeutic stance was of key importance. The **role of therapist in curiously working with the client to understand** embodied emotional experience and its meaning was considered crucial. This contrasted directly with a therapist making assumptions about emotions that only moved the client further from their understanding.

> *She'd say I know you're probably feeling this and that was kind of, like, just ... that would end up just being more confusing because then I kind of go, am I feeling that? I don't know whether I am, and then I think she knows better than me so ... I think just that kind of presumption that although you might know certain facts about someone, you can't necessarily say how they're feeling because that just pushes their feelings away.* (client participant)

This work appeared to reflect that, through the therapeutic relationship, it was important for emotion to be carefully explored, validated, connected with, followed, and made meaning of, to achieve an improved understanding of the self.

Identifying Relevant Psychotherapeutic Theory-based Methods of Change

Taken together, this development work enabled us to 'map' hypothesised change processes and associated mechanisms of change theorised to lead to the emergence and integration of an 'emotional self', described as the 'Real Me'. This process involved removing of blocks to access emotion which could then be identified, expressed, made meaning of, and processed, leading to a greater understanding and connection with the self. From here, psychotherapeutic intervention theory could then be applied to consider how psychotherapeutic practice may facilitate such change. This was explored in a consensus group of the authors of this book across six intervention development meetings.

During SPEAKS development meetings, routes/goals of change in different models were compared against identified descriptions/processes of change associated with recovery for people with AN. Several clinical models of *emotional processing* have been proposed with varying degrees of commonalities and difference and goals of working with emotion vary between psychotherapeutic models (Pascual-Leone, 2018). However, it is proposed that all psychotherapeutic models incorporate *subtypes* of 'emotional processing', including awareness, affective arousal, emotion regulation, and cognitive reflection on emotion (Pascual-Leone et al., 2016). For example, many clinical approaches recognise the importance of an ability to usefully regulate emotion (e.g. Dialetical Behaviour Therapy, CBT, and third wave approaches such as Acceptance and Commitment Therapy or Mindfulness Based Cognitive Therapy, Emotion Focused Therapy, Schema Therapy; Dadomo et al., 2016; Elliott & Greenberg, 2021; Hill & Updegraff, 2012; Neacsiu et al., 2014). Yet, our work informed us that how emotion regulation is approached is important and also that an ability to connect with, tolerate, trust, and use embodied emotional information was required.

Both Emotion Focused Therapy and Schema Therapy involve experientially connecting with, validating, making sense of, and processing emotional material via identifying and holding previously hidden important needs, leading to development of new meanings, narratives, and enhanced understanding of self, relationships, and the world (Lockwood & Samson, 2020; Paivio, 2013). Emphasised in Emotion Focused Therapy is the process of emotion transformation or 'changing emotion with emotion' as a route to resolve stuck emotional processes (e.g. persistent shame) that are driving symptomatic presentations (Greenberg & Pascual-Leone, 2024). Working with specific emotions such as shame, guilt, and loneliness were noted as significant in our development work. Furthermore, both Emotion Focused Therapy and Schema Therapy hold the therapeutic relationship as central to change which further aligned with reflections from those with lived experience. Emotion Focused Therapy and Schema Therapy were therefore considered highly relevant to the emotion change processes underpinning the emergence of the 'Real Me' identified in our development work as associated with recovery from anorexia.

Emotion Focused Therapy and Schema Therapy

Emotion Focused Therapy (EFT) is centred upon the role of emotion in human functioning, which is seen as key to therapeutic change. A major premise in EFT is the principle that: "you have to arrive at a place (emotion) before you can leave it" (Greenberg & Pascual-Leone, 2024). EFT development dates from the 1970s. It began integrating experiential therapeutic methods from Gestalt and other humanistic therapies, whilst holding the frame of a person-centered relationship in which emotion was privileged as a source of meaning, direction, and growth (Elliott et al., 2004). By considering clients' internal processes rather than placing a singular emphasis on core conditions (empathy, congruence, and unconditional positive regard), EFT aimed to generate a more 'efficient' change process. EFT developers conducted analysis of in-session processes to 'map out' 'patterns of change' (Greenberg, 1986). They developed a series of individual, empirically-supported, within session tasks, each targeting a key therapeutic goal, such as self-critical processes or interpersonal relationship difficulties. These tasks were structured and guided client's emotional processing towards identifying and processing unmet needs, specifically seeking to promote three key processes: (1) processing and transforming underdeveloped emotional responses frozen in earlier life (usually related to chronic unmet childhood needs) that did not evolve as the client matured into adulthood, (2) seeing emotion as valid and helpful, thereby utilising emotion's innate adaptive potential via connecting emotion to cognition, and (3) emotion regulation (Greenberg & Pascual-Leone, 2024). EFT incorporates contemporary emotion theory, affective neuroscience, dialectical constructivism, and current attachment theory and has developed process-oriented, disorder specific, time-limited therapy protocols which account for both within-session and across-therapy change. It has an evidence base for treating a range of mental health difficulties (Elliott et al., 2021).

Schema Therapy (ST) developed during the late 1980s/early 1990s (Young, 1990) and evolved in response to the needs of individuals with more complex presentations and unable to benefit from traditional approaches to therapy, most prototypically those with 'personality disorder'. It had its roots in Cognitive Behavioural Therapy (CBT) approaches, although its founder, Young, noted that individuals who had endured relational trauma often had an unstable sense of self and struggled to trust and attach sufficiently to a therapist and therefore were not a good fit for traditional CBT which assumed individuals could form secure attachments with therapists and had stable and enduring 'core beliefs'. Relational frameworks for responding to attachment needs (Bowlby et al., 1992) were considered of relevance and were later translated into ST relational mechanisms of change (Young et al., 2003). ST conceptualises difficulties emerging from 'early maladaptive schemas' (EMS) arising from the notion of universal primary 'needs' being chronically unmet and leading to constraints in perceptions and relating in the world. There are five proposed core emotional needs: "(1) Secure attachments to others; (2) Autonomy, competence, and sense of identity; (3) Freedom to express valid needs and emotions; (4) Spontaneity and play; (5) Realistic limits and self-control." (Young et al., 2003, p 10). ST thus takes an integrative psychotherapeutic approach and combines not only aspects of attachment therapies and CBT, but also psychodynamic and gestalt therapies. The evidence base for ST is most robust in treating 'Emotionally Unstable (Borderline) Personality Disorder' (Arntz et al., 2022; Arntz & Van Genderen, 2020; Rameckers et al., 2021).

Once these therapies were identified as relevant, their related theories further elucidated the SPEAKS model of change, and relevant therapeutic tasks and strategies to facilitate change in practice were reviewed, as discussed in Chapter 2, and elaborated throughout this guidebook.

References

Amianto, F., Northoff, G., Abbate Daga, G., Fassino, S., & Tasca, G. A. (2016). Is anorexia nervosa a disorder of the self? A psychological approach. *Frontiers in Psychology*, 7, 186132.

Arcelus, J., Haslam, M., Farrow, C., & Meyer, C. (2013). The role of interpersonal functioning in the maintenance of eating psychopathology: A systematic review and testable model. *Clinical Psychology Review*, 33(1), 156–167.

Arntz, A., Jacob, G. A., Lee, C. W., Brand-de Wilde, O. M., Fassbinder, E., Harper, R. P., Lavender, A., Lockwood, G., Malogiannis, I. A., & Ruths, F. A. (2022). Effectiveness of predominantly group schema therapy and combined individual and group schema therapy for borderline personality disorder: A randomized clinical trial. *JAMA Psychiatry*, *79*(4), 287–299.

Arntz, A., & Van Genderen, H. (2020). *Schema therapy for borderline personality disorder*. John Wiley & Sons.

Bardone-Cone, A. M., Hunt, R. A., & Watson, H. J. (2018). An overview of conceptualizations of eating disorder recovery, recent findings, and future directions. *Current Psychiatry Reports*, *20*, 1–18.

Bardone-Cone, A. M., Thompson, K. A., & Miller, A. J. (2020). The self and eating disorders. *Journal of Personality*, *88*(1), 59–75.

Barrett, L. F., Mesquita, B., Ochsner, K. N., & Gross, J. J. (2007). The experience of emotion. *Annual Review of Psychology*, *58*, 373–403.

Bowlby, J., Ainsworth, M., & Bretherton, I. (1992). The origins of attachment theory. *Developmental Psychology*, *28*(5), 759–775.

Braun, V., & Clarke, V. (2012). *Thematic analysis*. American Psychological Association.

Brockmeyer, T., Skunde, M., Wu, M., Bresslein, E., Rudofsky, G., Herzog, W., & Friederich, H.-C. (2014). Difficulties in emotion regulation across the spectrum of eating disorders. *Comprehensive Psychiatry*, *55*(3), 565–571.

Bruch, H. (1982). Anorexia Nervosa: Therapy and theory. *The American Journal of Psychiatry*, *139*(12), 1531–1538.

Croce, S. R., Malcolm, A. C., Ralph-Nearman, C., & Phillipou, A. (2024). The role of identity in anorexia nervosa: A narrative review. *New Ideas in Psychology*, *72*, 101060.

Dadomo, H., Grecucci, A., Giardini, I., Ugolini, E., Carmelita, A., & Panzeri, M. (2016). Schema therapy for emotional dysregulation: Theoretical implication and clinical applications. *Frontiers in Psychology*, *7*, 209621.

Damasio, A. (2003). Feelings of emotion and the self. *Annals of the New York Academy of Sciences*, *1001*(1), 253–261.

Davies, L., Griffiths, M. Lavender, T & Oldershaw, A. (in prep). Experiences of engaging with emotion and emotional change in recovery from anorexia nervosa: Learning from lived experience of people with anorexia, family members and therapists.

Dolhanty, J., & Greenberg, L. S. (2009). Emotion-focused therapy in a case of anorexia nervosa. *Clinical Psychology & Psychotherapy: An International Journal of Theory & Practice*, *16*(4), 336–382.

Drinkwater, D., Holttum, S., Lavender, T., Startup, H., & Oldershaw, A. (2022). Seeing through the façade of anorexia: A grounded theory of emotional change processes associated with recovery from anorexia nervosa. *Frontiers in Psychiatry*, 1316.

Elliott, R., & Greenberg, L. (2021). *Emotion-focused counselling in action*. Sage.

Elliott, R., Watson, J. C., Goldman, R. N., & Greenberg, L. S. (2004). *Learning emotion-focused therapy: The process-experiential approach to change*. American Psychological Association.

Elliott, R., Watson, J. C., Timulak, L., & Sharbanee, J. (2021). Research on humanistic-experiential psychotherapies: Updated review. *Bergin and Garfield's handbook of psychotherapy and behavior change*, 421–467.

Gaudio, S., Brooks, S. J., & Riva, G. (2014). Nonvisual multisensory impairment of body perception in anorexia nervosa: A systematic review of neuropsychological studies. *PloS one*, *9*(10), e110087.

Greenberg, L. S. (1986). Change process research. *Journal of Consulting and Clinical Psychology, 54*(1), 4.

Greenberg, L. S. (2004). Emotion–focused therapy. *Clinical Psychology & Psychotherapy: An International Journal of Theory & Practice, 11*(1), 3–16.

Greenberg, L. S., & Pascual-Leone, A. (2024). Changing emotion with emotion. In *Change in Emotion and Mental Health* (pp. 325–344). Elsevier.

Hatch, A., Madden, S., Kohn, M. R., Clarke, S., Touyz, S., Gordon, E., & Williams, L. M. (2010). Emotion brain alterations in anorexia nervosa: a candidate biological marker and implications for treatment. *Journal of Psychiatry and Neuroscience, 35*(4), 267–274.

Hill, C. L., & Updegraff, J. A. (2012). Mindfulness and its relationship to emotional regulation. *Emotion, 12*(1), 81–90.

Huke, V., Turk, J., Saeidi, S., Kent, A., & Morgan, J. F. (2013). Autism spectrum disorders in eating disorder populations: a systematic review. *European Eating Disorders Review, 21*(5), 345–351.

Karwautz, A., Völkl-Kernstock, S., Nobis, G., Kalchmayr, G., Hafferl-Gattermayer, A., Wöber-Bingöl, Ç., & Friedrich, M. H. (2001). Characteristics of self-regulation in adolescent patients with anorexia nervosa. *British Journal of Medical Psychology, 74*(1), 101–114.

Lavender, J. M., Wonderlich, S. A., Engel, S. G., Gordon, K. H., Kaye, W. H., & Mitchell, J. E. (2015). Dimensions of emotion dysregulation in anorexia nervosa and bulimia nervosa: A conceptual review of the empirical literature. *Clinical Psychology Review, 40*, 111–122.

Lockwood, G., & Samson, R. (2020). Understanding and meeting core emotional needs. In *Creative Methods in Schema Therapy* (pp. 76–90). Routledge.

Loureiro, F., Ringold, S. M., & Aziz-Zadeh, L. (2024). Interoception in autism: A narrative review of behavioral and neurobiological data. *Psychology Research and Behavior Management*, 1841–1853.

Monteleone, A. M., Cascino, G., Martini, M., Patriciello, G., Ruzzi, V., Delsedime, N., Abbate-Daga, G., & Marzola, E. (2021). Confidence in one-self and confidence in one's own body: The revival of an old paradigm for anorexia nervosa. *Clinical Psychology & Psychotherapy, 28*(4), 818–827.

Monteleone, A. M., Castellini, G., Ricca, V., Volpe, U., De Riso, F., Nigro, M., Zamponi, F., Mancini, M., Stanghellini, G., & Monteleone, P. (2017). Embodiment mediates the relationship between avoidant attachment and eating disorder psychopathology. *European Eating Disorders Review, 25*(6), 461–468.

Neacsiu, A. D., Bohus, M., & Linehan, M. M. (2014). Dialectical behavior therapy: An intervention for emotion dysregulation. *Handbook of Emotion Regulation, 2*, 491–507.

Oldershaw, A., Hambrook, D., Stahl, D., Tchanturia, K., Treasure, J., & Schmidt, U. (2011). The socio-emotional processing stream in anorexia nervosa. *Neuroscience & Biobehavioral Reviews, 35*(3), 970–988.

Oldershaw, A., Lavender, T., Sallis, H., Stahl, D., & Schmidt, U. (2015). Emotion generation and regulation in anorexia nervosa: a systematic review and meta-analysis of self-report data. *Clinical Psychology Review, 39*, 83–95.

Oldershaw, A., Lavender, T., & Schmidt, U. (2018). Are socio-emotional and neurocognitive functioning predictors of therapeutic outcomes for adults with anorexia nervosa? *European Eating Disorders Review, 26*(4), 346–359.

Oldershaw, A., Startup, H., & Lavender, T. (2019). Anorexia nervosa and a lost emotional self: a psychological formulation of the development, maintenance, and treatment of anorexia nervosa. *Frontiers in Psychology*, *10*, 219.

Paivio, S. C. (2013). Essential processes in emotion-focused therapy. *Psychotherapy*, *50*(3), 341.

Pascual-Leone, A. (2018). How clients "change emotion with emotion": A programme of research on emotional processing. *Psychotherapy Research*, *28*(2), 165–182.

Pascual-Leone, A., Paivio, S., & Harrington, S. (2016). Emotion in psychotherapy: An experiential–humanistic perspective. In D. J. Cain, K. Keenan, & S. Rubin (Eds.), *Humanistic psychotherapies: Handbook of research and practice* (2nd ed., pp. 147–181). American Psychological Association. https://doi.org/10.1037/14775-006.

Rameckers, S. A., Verhoef, R. E., Grasman, R. P., Cox, W. R., van Emmerik, A. A., Engelmoer, I. M., & Arntz, A. (2021). Effectiveness of psychological treatments for borderline personality disorder and predictors of treatment outcomes: a multivariate multilevel meta-analysis of data from all design types. *Journal of Clinical Medicine*, *10*(23), 5622.

Schmidt, U., & Treasure, J. (2014). The Maudsley Model of Anorexia Nervosa Treatment for Adults (MANTRA): Development, key features, and preliminary evidence. *Journal of Cognitive Psychotherapy*, *28*(1), 48–71.

Seth, A. K. (2013). Interoceptive inference, emotion, and the embodied self. *Trends in Cognitive Sciences*, *17*(11), 565–573.

Stanghellini, G., Mancini, M., Castellini, G., & Ricca, V. (2018). Eating disorders as disorders of embodiment and identity: Theoretical and empirical perspectives. In H. L. McBride & J. L. Kwee (Eds.), *Embodiment and eating disorders* (pp. 127–141). Routledge.

Stockford, C., Stenfert Kroese, B., Beesley, A., & Leung, N. (2019). Women's recovery from anorexia nervosa: A systematic review and meta-synthesis of qualitative research. *Eating Disorders*, *27*(4), 343–368.

Wildes, J. E., & Marcus, M. D. (2011). Development of emotion acceptance behavior therapy for anorexia nervosa: A case series. *International Journal of Eating Disorders*, *44*(5), 421–427.

Young, J. E. (1990). *Schema-focused cognitive therapy for personality disorders: A schema focused approach*. Professional Resource Exchange.

Young, J. E., Klosko, J. S., & Weishaar, M. E. (2003). *Schema therapy: A practitioner's guide*. Guilford Press.

Chapter 2

Theory and Conceptualisation of SPEAKS Therapy

The Specialist Psychotherapy with Emotion for Anorexia in Kent and Sussex (SPEAKS) approach understands emotions as learnt or instinctive responses to external or internal stimuli informing about our immediate environments, relationships, and crucially, our associated needs, thus guiding us towards action. This highlights the role of emotions as adaptive and useful. However, emotions are also reflective of our experience in life and will be influenced by this. This is particularly true of emotional states linked to unmet childhood needs and following ruptures in early co-regulation of emotion in the relationship with our primary caregiver, which go on to become "chronic self-defining emotions" (Timulak & Keogh, 2022, p 19). As such, some adults or adolescents are more easily triggered into certain emotional states which are linked to past unmet needs – such as abandonment, shame, or rage – even where they are not a good fit for the present situation. Therapy therefore requires increased connection with these early emotional states, but also making meaning of emotion to develop a nuanced understanding, a clear formulation of emotion, and knowledge of how and when emotional processing and emotional change is facilitated. Difficulties with emotion are evident in anorexia nervosa (AN) presentations (Oldershaw et al., 2015), and SPEAKS argues that emotion avoidance cycles and their impact upon the development and awareness of a core 'emotional self' are crucial foci for treatment, such that connection with and transformation of core painful stuck emotions generates the emergence of the 'Real Me', an integrated and coherent sense of self. In this chapter, we discuss this emotion theory in further depth and describe the emotion change process and research relevant to SPEAKS. We go on to outline and justify the emotion change processes targeted in SPEAKS therapy.

What Are Emotions?

Emotions, affect, mood, feelings are just some of the overarching frames and language we give to our internal experiences of emotional arousal. In evolutionary terms, emotions are deemed as having utility in our lives; they are the basis for construction and organisation of the Self. Emotion evolved to be experienced on both

DOI: 10.4324/9781003468349-3

physiological and psychological levels, affording rapid information processing which can be used to guide action based on personal needs, values, and goals. Each emotion is broadly associated with a different action tendency to meet immediate need (Elliott & Greenberg, 2021). For example, fear typically mobilises us to run away or to freeze, while anger pushes us to assert ourselves or attack. In infancy our emotions communicate to our primary caregiver what we need, guiding them to meet our needs and leading to co-regulation of emotion. Emotion is thus also a communication system, regulating the Self and others and giving life meaning and purpose (Greenberg, 2004).

Some therapeutic approaches or literature ascribe further values to emotion such as assigning categories of 'positive emotions' (e.g. joy, curiosity) and 'negative' emotions (e.g. anger, sadness, shame) dependent upon how pleasant or comfortable they are generally perceived to feel. Judging emotions in this broad brush way is problematic and can lead to development of beliefs that certain (negative) emotions should be avoided, hidden, and not expressed, resulting in the development or perpetuation of emotional avoidance cycles, like those noted to occur for people with anorexia. It contradicts with evolutionary understanding of emotions and can result in us missing important information about ourselves and our needs. Furthermore, suppressed or avoided feelings don't ameliorate, rather they intensify, and unregulated, ignored emotions can become buried (alive) without an outlet.

Literature about emotions can also assign labels of basic or primary emotions (simple and immediate such as anger or joy) and secondary or complex emotions (requiring and based in self-reflection and cognitive evaluation such as guilt or pride). SPEAKS therapy bases its understanding of emotion in evolutionary psychology and Emotion Focused Therapy (EFT) theory. As such, emotions are not classified as 'positive' or 'negative', rather they are seen as adaptive or maladaptive depending on the context in which they arise, and primary or secondary depending on the proximity of their relationship to the trigger (Greenberg, 2004). It is important to note that with this understanding all emotions can be described as adaptive or maladaptive and primary or secondary since this is situation dependent and not an intrinsic feature of each emotion itself.

Primary Adaptive Emotion

A primary emotion that is adaptive is one which arises as a direct response to what happens in a situation. It is new, 'fresh', and informs us of our immediate need and the appropriate related action to take. For example, *primary adaptive* sadness over the loss of someone or something important to us can tell us that we need comfort and connection, leading us to cry out and reach for closeness with another, be that physically (e.g. a hug) and/or emotionally (e.g. sharing and describing our pain with a trusted other). By meeting the need in this way, our sadness is regulated and reduced. Although our sadness can still be present to some degree, we may now also feel additional emotion, such as warmth and calm.

Primary Maladaptive Emotion: Core Pain of Unmet Needs

Human emotions become complex multicomponent phenomena over time with increased life experience. Lived emotional experience arises from a complex synthesis of many processes, starting from innate biologically driven building blocks (e.g. temperament, genetics) and later incorporating cognitive, memory, motivational, and behavioural data (Greenberg et al., 2024). Therefore, sometimes, our immediate emotional reaction to a situation is not related to our here-and-now experiences but rather to old feelings related to past experiences, particularly in relation to developmental needs that were chronically unmet. These are our *emotional ghosts from the past* or "chronic self-defining emotions" (Timulak & Keogh, 2022, p 19).

These persistent and chronic emotions become our emotional vulnerabilities. In EFT they are known as *primary maladaptive emotions*, with core pain being the primary maladaptive emotion that hurts the most (Timulak & Keogh, 2022). In SPEAKS, we use the terms primary maladaptive emotions and core pain interchangeably, favouring the term core pain. These core painful feelings are often described as stuck feelings and are extremely familiar to clients. Core pain is experienced even in new situations for which it is a poor fit, rendering it unhelpful and fruitless in identifying and meeting current needs. Core pain encompasses past needs that were chronically unmet and resultant core schemata (such as defectiveness, abandonment, emotional deprivation). Unmet needs can cover a range of domains, with Schema Therapy (ST) outlining five main types (Young et al., 2003), and which here we cluster into three broad groups, although it should be noted that idiosyncrasies remain (Timulak & Keogh, 2022).

First, unmet attachment needs, such as a need for love, connection, and closeness with loved ones are associated with painful emotions of loneliness or sadness. Secondly, unmet needs associated with identity formation such as needs for acceptance, respect, acknowledgement, and understanding are associated with feelings such as shame. Thirdly are unmet needs for safety, that is for protection, control, and comfort, and which can include the safety to be myself, such as to express valid needs and emotions and for spontaneity and play. Unmet safety needs are associated with fear-based emotions.

A child with unmet identity needs of feeling accepted, valued, and appreciated can internalise the message "There is something defective and wrong with me" (defectiveness schema) and experience a core pain of shame. Later in life, that core pain becomes easily triggered, even where it is not relevant to the situation at hand. Shame for example can be quickly experienced in relation to any real or presumed insult or disapproval, even when relatively benign or small. This can result in hiding away or becoming submissive. This may have been appropriate at one point in the past (e.g. to keep safe) or been the only available response for a child within the context. However, as an adult, this learnt ill-fitting response blocks adaptive emotions and helpful action, such as positive problem-solving or standing up for ourselves, thus interfering with healthy functioning. Core pain perpetuates learnt unhelpful inter- and intra-personal relationship patterns, impeding personal growth and agency. It is linked to a range of symptomatic mental health presentations (Timulak & Keogh, 2022). As such, core pain is a key target for treatment in EFT, ST, and SPEAKS.

Secondary Emotion

Sometimes we are unaware of an experience of primary emotions because they are very quickly 'covered up' or hidden by a secondary emotion rendering the primary emotion beyond our current conscious awareness (Greenberg, 2010). Secondary emotions are usually protective in nature, disconnecting us from vulnerable painful feelings, typically core pain, although they can also protect against painful adaptive primary emotions that we find difficult to accept or face. An example of this is anger leading to someone lashing out in response to a triggering of shame beyond our consciousness. We might describe it as humiliated fury, a rage covering a primary maladaptive core pain of shame linked to past unmet needs around validation and acknowledgement. Such secondary emotion is usually disproportionately intense and not well-regulated. Following action tendencies of secondary anger such as setting boundaries or 'puffing up' in relation to another person may in the short-term improve sense of relative worth and lead to a reduction in overall emotion. However, it does not ultimately resolve the underlying core issues of shame which will continue to persist, hidden and unrecognised.

Triggers of and Blocks to Core Pain

Clients usually attend therapy as a result of a range of symptomatic presentations. For people with eating disorders (EDs), they may present on the surface with distress arising from the self-comparisons and harsh self-criticism associated with trying to achieve a particular body or harmful eating behaviours. Triggers are usually based in an historical context associated with painful (often interpersonal) experiences (e.g. bullying around weight/shape) but interact with present day events (e.g. a perceived disgusted facial expression or comment from a close other) resulting in increased symptomatology and self-criticism and patterns of unhelpful coping to manage emotional pain. Furthermore, where individuals have endured trauma, all emotions may become associated with threat.

Ways of coping with core pain can involve behaviours such as avoiding emotion, keeping people at arm's length, or high levels of cognitive distraction, but they can be more fully understood as complex moment-to-moment temporary states or 'modes' (Young et al., 2003). These modes reflect a 'part of the self' which encompasses not just a behaviour, but a cluster of emotions, action tendencies, physiological experiences and cognitions, associated with past memories and experiences (overlapping with the concept of Emotion Schemes in EFT; Greenberg, 2010). For example, secondary emotion of anger associated with action tendencies such as 'puffing up' in aggression and pushing others away physically/metaphorically to protect from underlying core pain, alongside physiological experiences such as a flushed face and raised blood pressure and cognitions like, "This other person is treating me badly because they do not respect me. It is all their fault." We might call this an Angry Protector 'part of self' utilised to cope (Keulen-de Vos et al., 2016). Indeed, it is argued that we might all move between a range of 'parts of self' to cope in life – each reflecting a specific constellation of feelings, thoughts, physiological experiences, action tendencies and episodic memories – and thus we are each a product of our own self-multiplicity, where we are composed of many interacting 'parts' (Pugh, 2021). These different parts or 'modes' of being are our best attempts to manage life, and they may be more or less helpful, depending on the strategies we were taught by primary caregivers and learnt for ourselves across life experiences.

In ST 'parts of self' include coping modes, critic parts, and child parts. In EFT, these are thought of as coaches, critics, guards, or experiencers. In either case, a part of self can be a constant trigger of core pain (e.g. critic) or a way to avoid and cope with core pain (e.g. coping modes). This prevents us from accessing our primary emotions (whether adaptive or maladaptive) and thus is a block to, or interrupter of, useful emotion processing. Utilising ST and EFT, SPEAKS applies a model of self-multiplicity to seek to understand how an individual learnt to cope with their core pain, how this impacted the development of the Self, the costs of this way of managing and how it prevents access to adaptive emotional experience and future personal growth. This approach considers the whole person; it values and privileges an understanding of how the Self is developed and how 'parts of self' interact.

Inner Critic

The concept of an 'Inner Critic' refers to a system of critical and negative thoughts and attitudes towards the Self that interfere with a person's experiencing process. It is similar to concepts described in other psychotherapeutic approaches, such as 'harsh superego' in psychoanalysis, a 'critical parent' in transactional analysis or earlier accounts of ST, 'top dog' in Gestalt therapy and 'negative self-critical thoughts' in cognitive-behavioural therapy (Stinckens et al., 2013). We all have an internal voice which at the milder end can resemble a critic which keeps us in check and helps us to function. At the more extreme end, individuals endure harsh punitive or guilt-inducing internal critical dialogues, sometimes with the qualities/ tone of (an) actual person(s) from earlier in their life (e.g. abusive parent or bully). Thus self-criticism arises from schemata about the Self, formed as a consequence of chronic unmet need (Young et al. 2003). The Inner Critic espouses judgements about one's characterological flaws in self-defining terms internalised as first-person statements ("I am useless.", "I am a bad person.") (Timulak & Keogh, 2021). Such statements are usually perceived by people entering therapy as the 'truth' about who they are and therefore right and deserved, regardless of how harsh.

A strong Inner Critic that is punitive and demanding is characteristic of EDs (Simpson et al., 2018; Stinckens et al., 2013). For people with AN, an additional part emerges reflecting ED thoughts, the strength of which is related to ED psychopathology (Pugh & Waller, 2016). The form of the Eating Disorder Part (EDP) changes over time as the ED develops. At first the EDP is experienced as positive and congenial, an affiliate relationship, in which the EDP is seen as supportive, helpful, and enabling the client to meet their needs (Pugh, 2020). In this stage it may have more of a 'coaching' tone to its presentation. However, over time the EDP becomes increasingly hostile, coercive, and dominant (Pugh, 2020). It is punitive and undermines self-esteem. Now it demands unrelenting standards, with perfectionism and achievement focused on the body and eating/exercise behaviours (Simpson et al., 2018). As such, it represents both a means of protection from core pain and a contributing factor to its perpetuation.

Coping Modes

Understandably, people will develop ways to appease or quieten the critical part of self and to protect themself from core pain. The experiencing states comprised of behavioural patterns, cognitive processes, and emotional responses which seek to protect from core pain are known in ST as coping modes (Edwards, 2022) and in EFT as coaches or guards (Elliott et al., 2004). Coping modes are adaptive at the time of development (in childhood), often essential to survival, yet they may be over-relied upon and too stringent in their methods for optimum well-being in adulthood. Ultimately they are all parts of self which have the potential to interrupt the accessing and processing of useful emotional material.

Our early experiences and chronic unmet needs develop the 'lenses' (pervasive themes or schemata) through which we make sense of ourselves and the motivations and intentions of others, organising subsequent behaviour to best cope with and navigate the world around us (Lavender & Startup, 2018). Thus 'coping modes' develop alongside core pain in the context of life experiences and chronic unmet needs as our best attempts to cope with persistent painful experiences. Coping modes therefore reflect a desire to appease or quieten the critical part of self and/or can arise as a means to protect from underlying core pain. For example, early life experiences such as being emotionally overwhelmed and burdened by the needs of a parent results in chronically unmet attachment needs for love, connection, and closeness and can impede attunement and free expression of one's own emotions and internal experiences. This leads to a chronic sense of isolation linked to the sadness and loneliness of a a core pain of abandonment fears (lonely abandonment), which can be expressed as "I feel on my own" or "I have nobody to turn to." In such circumstances, attuning to the parent's emotional needs and meeting the needs of the parent may have gone some way to get attachment needs met and to feel (albeit fluctuating and conditional) closeness with the parent. Navigating the situation in this way will have led to development of coping strategies in 'modes' such as surrendering to and prioritising the needs of the parent which later becomes generalised to other relationships ('People Pleaser' mode or 'Compliant Surrenderer'). Such experiences are likely to be associated with the development of beliefs that one's own emotions and needs are unnecessary or of no value, further resulting in the development of parts which interrupt emotional experience and process through avoidance and 'numbing' of emotion ('Detached Protector' mode) or supressing emotion through compensatory coping modes (e.g. linked to behaviours such as worry, procrastination).

Coping modes are often associated with secondary emotional states, such as the secondary rage that pushes others away in a coping mode of Angry Protector to guard against experiencing the agonising core pain of shame. A coping mode of 'perfectionism', a trait commonly associated with AN (Edwards, 2017), protects against a core pain of chronic shame by attempting to prove one is worthy, leading to self-coercion reflecting overcompensation, overcontrolling, and setting high and unrelenting standards in an attempt never to 'fail'. Coping modes noted to be especially representative of eating disorder populations are 'Helpless Surrenderer' (self-neglect, giving in, and depending on others entirely for rescue or care, such as seeking hospitalisation so that the decision to eat is no longer theirs to make), 'Detached Self-soother' (cutting off from and interrupting emotion using distracting and unhelpful soothing behaviours, including ED behaviours such as excessive exercise or binging) and 'Compliant Surrenderer' (people-pleasing and meeting other's needs, even at the persistent expense of one's own) (Simpson et al., 2018).

Simpson and colleagues (2018) conceptualise the EDP as a coping mode rather than a critic. This can be particularly true in the earlier stages of the relationship where it is presenting more benignly as a perfectionist or coach. In SPEAKS, we see the EDP as straddling both a role of critic and coping mode. We frame the EDP within the critic conceptualisation, in part because of its close link to the broader Inner Critic and its role in the process of therapeutic change as a means to access the broader critic. That said, the EDP is perceived in SPEAKS to have a very close and entangled relationship with coping modes, where it can be seen to bolster or enhance the effectiveness of different ways of coping. For example, the behavioural range of a Detached Self-soother is expanded by excessive exercise or binging. The perfectionist overcontroller has more to focus on and more ways to achieve when calories and weight loss become additional means to overcompensate. Indeed, the frequency of many coping modes is positively correlated with ED symptoms, reflecting their inter-related nature (Simpson et al., 2018). This merging of the EDP across 'parts of self' is one of the reasons why EDs such as AN become so entrenched and complex over time as they intertwine with many aspects of functioning, and they become integral to a person's sense of self and identity.

It is useful to note that we all operate via coping modes at times. They are strategies by which we manage daily life. Coping modes can reflect our strengths too and enable us to flourish where the environment matches our primary ways of coping. However, coping modes which are overused can keep someone stuck and crucially disconnected from authentic emotions and needs. If coping modes become too stable over time they become default modes, appearing to reflect a stable personality (Lobbestael, 2007), but disconnected from adaptive feelings and needs. Conversely, dysregulated clients may very quickly move or 'flip' between modes making it difficult for the therapist to track their presenting state within sessions (Kellogg & Young, 2006). In this way people get caught in vicious cycles within and across modes, moving one continually further from their 'emotional self'. Thus, SPEAKS therapy seeks to help people understand their parts of self and how they relate, enabling them to reduce reliance on coping modes in order to bypass these blocks to experience and facilitate connection with adaptive emotions and needs.

Core Pain as a Focus for SPEAKS Therapy

Accessing Core Pain

Secondary emotion is often encountered in the early stages of therapy, captured in the surface narrative of 'presenting problems' and linked to coping modes. Our development work and the clinical literature indicates that people with AN usually enter therapy with global distress, anxiety, and some degree of guilt or disgust about their physical appearance and weight, connected with a harsh EDP, resulting in symptomatic behaviours and a range of coping modes to manage. This presentation is important in that it represents the person's current emotional state and provides valuable information as to coping modes at play and the strength of the eating disorder and internal critic; it requires attunement and validation. Connecting with secondary emotions and associated *coping modes*, however, is seen as a means to understand and move beyond them in order to connect to and engage with core pain and associated unmet needs. In SPEAKS, core pain is seen as housed in a part of self we call the '*Little Self*' which reflects the early childhood origins of its experience and the developmental unmet needs attached (this is known in ST as the 'Vulnerable Child' and in EFT as the 'Experiencing Self' in child mode; Oldershaw & Startup, 2020).

The most strongly reported schemata by people with anorexia are *defectiveness and shame* ("I am unloveable and broken"), *social isolation* ("I am alone"), and *subjugation* ("My feelings aren't important. It is not safe to be myself") (Oldershaw et al., 2015). This alongside commonly expressed emotions of abandonment and worthlessness (Dolhanty & Greenberg, 2007), indicates core pain encompassing themes of both chronically unmet identity needs and attachment needs, with some unmet safety needs. Whilst the EDP will have first appeared as a way to 'fix' what is 'defective' and 'broken' by promising a solution to potential rejection, i.e. meeting unmet identity needs (Burnett-Stuart et al., 2024), over time it will become increasingly harsh and hostile (Pugh, 2020). Instead of relieving unmet need and countering associated early beliefs, these will instead become perpetuated and strengthened by a now harsh and critical EDP. This only leads to engagement in further eating disorder behaviours (connected with coping modes such as Detached

Protector and People Pleaser) to appease and avoid the EDP and associated core pain. In SPEAKS, the core pain is thus hypothesised to be primarily both shame-based and linked to unmet identity needs, alongside the loneliness and sadness of abandonment fears (lonely abandonment) arising from unmet attachment needs.

This core pain can be understood to have developed in a connected pattern. Core pain of lonely abandonment and sadness reflects unmet needs of emotional valid-ation, closeness, connection, or caring internalised as "I am alone; I have nobody to turn to; Nobody wants to hear or can help me manage my emotions." There is a pervasive sense of being undeserving of the closeness and connection craved, lead-ing to conclusions that there must be a good reason for this and inciting internalisa-tions that, "I am unlovable, broken and defective", connected with shame (unmet identity needs) and a broad sense of anxiety or fear ("It is not safe to be myself"). Over time the EDP can itself come to represent an introjected attachment figure (Forsén Mantilla et al., 2019); now the possibility of moving on from the EDP in AN recovery further triggers the experience of core pain of abandonment associ-ated schemata, contributing to pervasiveness and stuckness.

Transforming Core Pain

Important to emotional change in SPEAKS are key principles of emotion processing including awareness, expression, regulation, and reflection (Pascual-Leone, 2018). New meanings are made through experiencing of emotion (Greenberg & Angus, 2004) and by understanding emotional patterns, ways of relating, and ways of cop-ing. Further to this, essential processes for therapeutic change include those which transform core painful emotions (Greenberg & Pascual-Leone, 2024). Emotion transformation is facilitated by connection with (developmental) unmet needs and by accessing and articulating what core pain needs/needed to locate associ-ated and useful primary adaptive emotion (Greenberg et al., 2024; Figure 2.1). The client becomes engaged in *productive expression* of previously constricted or hidden primary maladaptive emotions (Greenberg & Pascual-Leone, 2024) leading to transformation via coactivation of emotional states and their action tendencies, to synthesise new emotional experiences, meanings, and responses (Greenberg & Pascual-Leone, 2024). One cannot simultaneously hide in shame and thrust for-ward in productive anger that needs were not met, thereby the co-activation of the emotions and their action tendencies leads to a novel response and a transformed state, such as self-compassion. This process of accessing adaptive emotion whilst core pain is co-activated develops new narratives that can assimilate into and update existing cognitive structures. Thus, change occurs to both emotional experi-ence and the narratives in which they are embedded (Greenberg & Angus, 2004).

In the emotion transformation process, attention is given both to the emotion being reduced and to what emerges in its place. It rests upon the knowledge that there is no absence of emotion; processing one emotion to completion gives rise to a new changing experience emerging in its place (Gendlin, 1981). This said, emotion is also not transformed by simply seeking to *replace or add* one feeling to

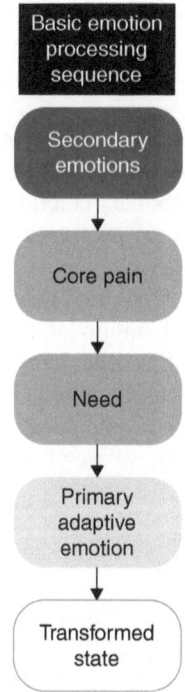

Figure 2.1 The Emotion Focused Therapy model of emotion change and transformation (adapted from (Greenberg et al., 2024; Pascual-Leone, 2018)

another or by focusing on preferred emotional states. The change process is contingent upon the emergence of the new synthesised experience from the repeated and
sustained co-activation of core pain and adaptive emotion that is transformative; it
is not simply a reduction of the old, core painful emotional experience.

Emotion transformation hinges in part upon 'memory reconsolidation' which
is a common transformational change process across psychotherapy approaches
(Ecker & Bridges, 2020). Memory reconsolidation involves uprooting problematic
memory structures and integrating new emotional information such that old episodic and autobiographical memories are updated (Goldman & Fredrick-Keniston,
2020). This mechanism of emotional change is explicitly utilised in both ST and
EFT, through experiential and imagery work (Arntz, 2012; Greenberg & Pascual-
Leone, 2024). It is further partly facilitated by a 'corrective emotional experience'
broadly considered a therapeutically powerful mechanism of therapeutic action
(Christian et al., 2012). The corrective emotional experience is a reliving of past
experiences in the present with a different and more positive emotional, relational,
cognitive, or behavioural impact and outcome. In psychotherapy sessions, this
occurs in the context of the therapeutic relationship breaking negative interpersonal

patterns and affording opportunities for emotional co-regulation which can be internalised and, ultimately, develop client emotion regulation capacity. The corrective emotional experience mechanism is central to EFT and ST (Greenberg, 2014; Gülüm & Soygüt, 2022).

This transformation model of sequential emotion change described is empirically demonstrated and associated with positive outcomes for therapy (Pascual-Leone, 2018). During 'working' (middle) phases of therapy, fewer secondary emotion and greater primary adaptive emotions significantly predict clinical outcomes from depression (Herrmann et al., 2016). Greater expression of primary adaptive emotion in particular leads to better outcomes (Herrmann et al., 2016), and this finding is reflected in our SPEAKS trial during which we tracked emotional change. We found that those who had 'good' outcomes (weight and ED behaviours both in the 'normal range' at the end of therapy) expressed significantly more primary adaptive emotion overall than those who did not change ('poor' outcomes), with this between-group difference emerging in the middle (working) phase of therapy (Malik-Smith et al., in prep).

SPEAKS Hypothesised Model of Emotion Change

SPEAKS holds at its core the sequential emotion change process (Pascual-Leone, 2018), informed by its programme of development work alongside EFT and ST theory and practice (Figure 2.2). Here we outline the application of the theory described to the presentation of AN in SPEAKS therapy. The most commonly reported emotions associated with change for people with AN are indicated; however, it is important to note that complexity of presentations and idiosyncrasies of people's lives will mean that actual emotions encountered and processed may vary widely, especially where there are multiple presentations at play.

In the early stages of therapy, secondary emotion is most often encountered. The EDP will be highly active at this stage, fuelling means of coping and associated emotions. This is captured in the surface narrative of 'presenting problems' and evident in global distress and guilt, self-disgust, or shame pertaining to the eating disorder. Secondary emotion housed in *coping modes* will be arising in response to core pain (e.g. feeling angry in response to shame; coping mode of Angry Protector) or covering it (e.g. guilt and disgust pertaining to the body/eating covering shame related to characterological aspects of the Self). This secondary emotion represents the person's current emotional state and provides valuable information as to coping modes at play and strength of the Inner Critic; it requires attunement and validation. Connecting with secondary emotions and associated coping modes, however, is seen as a means to understand and move beyond them to access core pain.

Engaging with the core pain of the Little Self represents a powerful change opportunity in the process of emotion transformation facilitated by connection with core pain and associated (developmental) unmet needs. By locating and experiencing core pain (e.g. lonely abandonment) and accessing the need inherent within it (e.g., being heard and emotionally connected/validated), clients can connect with

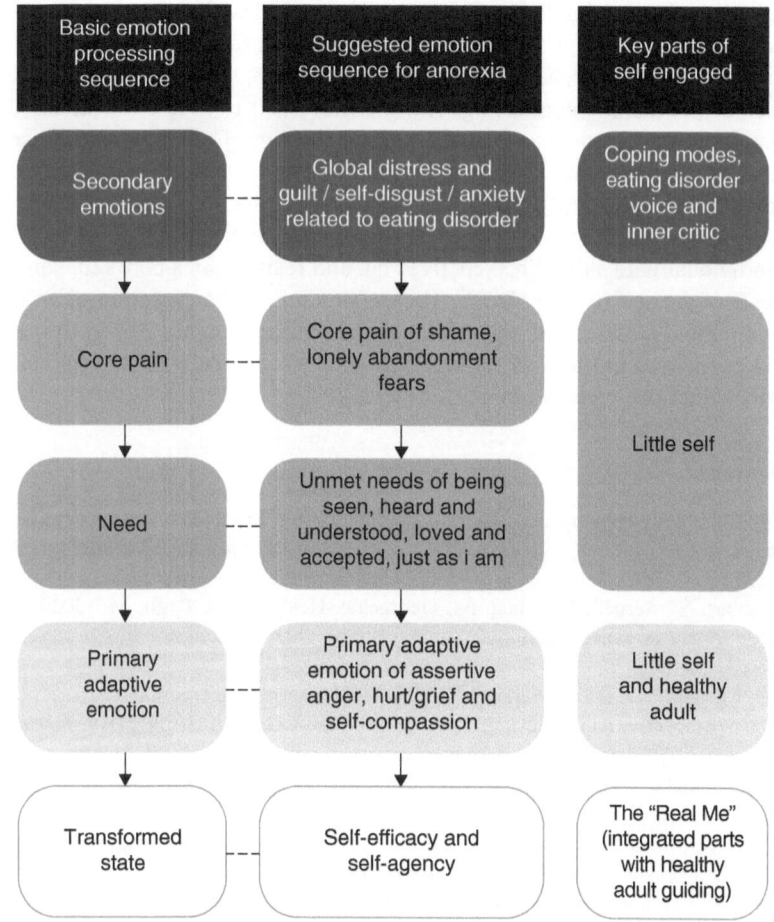

Figure. 2.2 The SPEAKS hypothesised model of emotional change and prevalence of parts of self during SPEAKS

vulnerability and move to discover and experience primary adaptive emotions and to process and make use of associated emotional information (e.g., grief and assertive anger that these needs were not met). In SPEAKS, we have identified that connecting with core painful shame, but then further accessing underlying loneliness/sadness-based core pain and its associated unmet needs, is important to the change process.

The co-activation of core pain and adaptive emotion leads to novel responses such as self-compassion and new narratives of the Self (e.g. "I deserved to have my needs met. I am not broken.") that can assimilate into existing schemata and cognitive structures and generate new ones. Specifically, from this emotion transformation process the 'functional' '*Healthy Adult*' can emerge characterised by the experience of adaptive emotions affording self-care and self-compassion (positive treatment of Self). Once a sufficient Healthy Adult is in play, clients can more readily identify, moderate, and move past coping modes, secondary emotions, and the Inner Critic, thereby connecting with the Little Self to access useful emotion information and to regulate and soothe painful feelings. Thus, a core premise of this way of working is that removing blocks to emotion and 'following the pain' to connect with what hurts the most and associated unmet need generates emotion transformation. This ultimately leads to subsequent growth and self-reorganisation of the individual with shifted persepctives on, and relationships between, some or all aspects of the self (e.g. the EDP). These shifts reflect the evolution of an integrated emotional sense of self – the 'Real Me' (Drinkwater et al., 2022). The 'Real Me' moves forward in life with self-agency and self-efficacy, no longer reliant on the EDP in attempts to get needs met.

References

Arntz, A. (2012). Imagery rescripting as a therapeutic technique: Review of clinical trials, basic studies, and research agenda. *Journal of Experimental Psychopathology*, *3*(2), 189–208.

Burnett-Stuart, S., Serpell, L., Chua, N., Georgeaux-Healy, C., & Pugh, M. (2024). The anorexic voice: A dialogical enquiry and thematic analysis. *Journal of Constructivist Psychology*, 1–20.

Christian, C., Safran, J. D., & Muran, J. C. (2012). The corrective emotional experience: A relational perspective and critique. In L. G. Castonguay & C. E. Hill (Eds.), *Transformation in psychotherapy: Corrective experiences across cognitive behavioral, humanistic, and psychodynamic approaches* (pp. 51–67). American Psychological Association. https://doi.org/10.1037/13747-004.

Dolhanty, J., & Greenberg, L. S. (2007). Emotion-focused therapy in the treatment of eating disorders. *European Psychotherapy*, *7*(1), 97–116.

Drinkwater, D., Holttum, S., Lavender, T., Startup, H., & Oldershaw, A. (2022). Seeing through the façade of anorexia: A grounded theory of emotional change processes associated with recovery from anorexia nervosa. *Frontiers in Psychiatry*, 1316.

Ecker, B., & Bridges, S. K. (2020). How the science of memory reconsolidation advances the effectiveness and unification of psychotherapy. *Clinical Social Work Journal*, *48*(3), 287–300. https://doi.org/10.1007/s10615-020-00754-z.

Edwards, D. J. (2017). An interpretative phenomenological analysis of schema modes in a single case of anorexia nervosa: Part 2. Coping modes, healthy adult mode, superordinate themes, and implications for research and practice. *Indo-Pacific Journal of Phenomenology*, *17*(1).

Edwards, D. J. A. (2022). Using schema modes for case conceptualization in schema therapy: An applied clinical approach [review]. *Frontiers in psychology*, *12*. https://doi.org/10.3389/fpsyg.2021.763670.

Elliott, R., & Greenberg, L. (2021). *Emotion-focused counselling in action*. Sage.

Elliott, R., Watson, J. C., Goldman, R. N., & Greenberg, L. S. (2004). *Learning emotion-focused therapy: The process-experiential approach to change*. American Psychological Association.

Forsén Mantilla, E., Clinton, D., & Birgegård, A. (2019). The unsafe haven: Eating disorders as attachment relationships. *Psychology and Psychotherapy: Theory, Research and Practice*, *92*(3), 379–393.

Gendlin, E. (1981). *Focusing*. Bantam.

Goldman, R., & Fredrick-Keniston, A. (2020). Memory reconsolidation as a common change process. In L. Nadel & R. D. Lane (Eds.) *Neuroscience of enduring change: Implications for psychotherapy* (pp. 328–359). Oxford University Press.

Greenberg, L. S. (2004). Emotion–focused therapy. *Clinical Psychology & Psychotherapy: An International Journal of Theory & Practice*, *11*(1), 3–16.

Greenberg, L. (2014). The therapeutic relationship in emotion-focused therapy. *Psychotherapy*, *51*(3), 350.

Greenberg, L., Pascual-Leone, J., & Johnson, J. (2024). Schematic processing and emotional change: Implications for treatment. *New Ideas in Psychology*, *73*, 101075.

Greenberg, L. S. (2010). Emotion-focused therapy: A clinical synthesis. *Focus*, *8*(1), 32–42.

Greenberg, L. S., & Angus, L. E. (2004). The contributions of emotion processes to narrative change in psychotherapy: A dialectical constructivist approach. In L. E. Angus & J. McLeod (Eds.), *The handbook of narrative and psychotherapy: Practice, theory, and research* (pp. 331–349). Sage Publications, Inc. https://doi.org/10.4135/9781412973496.d25.

Greenberg, L. S., & Pascual-Leone, A. (2024). Changing emotion with emotion. In A. C. Samson, D. Sander, U. Kramer (Eds.) *Change in Emotion and Mental Health* (pp. 325–344). Elsevier.

Gülüm, İ. V., & Soygüt, G. (2022). Limited reparenting as a corrective emotional experience in schema therapy: A preliminary task analysis. *Psychotherapy Research*, *32*(2), 263–276.

Herrmann, I. R., Greenberg, L. S., & Auszra, L. (2016). Emotion categories and patterns of change in experiential therapy for depression. *Psychotherapy Research*, *26*(2), 178–195.

Kellogg, S. H., & Young, J. E. (2006). Schema therapy for borderline personality disorder. *Journal of Clinical Psychology*, *62*(4), 445–458.

Keulen-de Vos, M. E., Bernstein, D. P., Vanstipelen, S., de Vogel, V., Lucker, T. P., Slaats, M., Hartkoorn, M., & Arntz, A. (2016). Schema modes in criminal and violent behaviour of forensic cluster B PD patients: A retrospective and prospective study. *Legal and Criminological Psychology*, *21*(1), 56–76.

Lavender, A., & Startup, H. (2018). Personality disorders. In S. Moorey & A. Lavender (Eds.) *The Therapeutic Relationship in Cognitive Behavioural Therapy* (pp. 174–188). SAGE.

Lobbestael, J., van Vreeswijk, M. & Arntz, A. (2007). Shedding light on schema modes: a clarification of the mode concept and its current research status. *NEJP, 63*, 69–78.

Malik-Smith, S., Papastavrou Brooks., C., Callanan, M., Pascual-Leone, A. & Oldershaw, A. (in prep) The process of emotion change associated with recovery from anorexia nervosa.

Oldershaw, A., Lavender, T., Sallis, H., Stahl, D., & Schmidt, U. (2015). Emotion generation and regulation in anorexia nervosa: A systematic review and meta-analysis of self-report data. *Clinical Psychology Review*, *39*, 83–95.

Oldershaw, A., & Startup, H. (2020). Building the healthy adult in eating disorders: A schema mode and emotion-focused therapy approach for anorexia nervosa. In G. Heath & H. Startup (Eds.) *Creative methods in schema therapy* (pp. 287–300). Routledge.

Pascual-Leone, A. (2018). How clients "change emotion with emotion": A programme of research on emotional processing. *Psychotherapy Research*, *28*(2), 165–182.

Pugh, M. (2020). Understanding "Ed": A theoretical and empirical review of the internal eating disorder "voice".. *BPS Psychother Sect Rev, 65*, 12–23.

Pugh, M. (2021). Single-session chairwork: overview and case illustration of brief dialogical psychotherapy. *British Journal of Guidance & Counselling*, 1–19.

Pugh, M., & Waller, G. (2016). The anorexic voice and severity of eating pathology in anorexia nervosa. *International Journal of Eating Disorders, 49*(6), 622–625.

Simpson, S. G., Pietrabissa, G., Rossi, A., Seychell, T., Manzoni, G. M., Munro, C., Nesci, J. B., & Castelnuovo, G. (2018). Factorial structure and preliminary validation of the Schema Mode Inventory for Eating Disorders (SMI-ED). *Frontiers in Psychology, 9*, 314057.

Stinckens, N., Lietaer, G., & Leijssen, M. (2013). Working with the inner critic: Process features and pathways to change. *Person-centered & Experiential Psychotherapies, 12*(1), 59–78.

Timulak, L., & Keogh, D. (2022). *Transdiagnostic emotion-focused therapy: A clinical guide for transforming emotional pain*. American Psychological Association.

Young, J. E., Klosko, J. S., & Weishaar, M. E. (2003). *Schema therapy: A practitioner's guide*. Guilford.

Chapter 3

Testing SPEAKS

Specialist Psychotherapy with Emotion for Anorexia in Kent and Sussex (SPEAKS) was developed in a programme of research comprised of two phases and conducted over six years. As outlined in Chapters 1 and 2, the first of these phases – SPEAKS Intervention Development – involved learning from people with lived experience about what had facilitated emotional change related to recovery and then applying psychological and psychotherapeutic theory to generate a model of how best to facilitate that change in psychological therapy. The current chapter will focus on the second phase of the SPEAKS research programme – Testing SPEAKS. It outlines feasibility trial findings, including the acceptability of SPEAKS and signals of efficacy. It goes on to describe a range of change process research studies designed to test the SPEAKS hypotheses of change.

Feasibility Trial

The feasibility trial (Oldershaw et al., 2024) was conducted within two UK National Health Service (NHS) outpatient specialist eating disorders services: Kent and Medway All Age Eating Disorder Service, North-East London NHS Foundation Trust, and Sussex Eating Disorder Service, Sussex Partnership NHS Foundation Trust. Consecutive referrals to the services that met inclusion criteria were approached for participation in the research and informed consent obtained. SPEAKS was delivered weekly over 9 to 12 months with the majority of sessions being conducted via online video platform due to the Covid-19 pandemic.

Participants

There were 34 participants in the SPEAKS feasibility trial. People who took part were predominantly White British (73.5%) females (97.0%). The average age at time of recruitment was 29 years. Eating disorder (ED) thoughts and behaviours were measured using the Eating Disorder Examination Questionnaire (EDEQ; Fairburn & Beglin, 2008), and the mean global score at baseline was 4.14 (sd = 1.1)

DOI: 10.4324/9781003468349-4

out of a maximum score of 6, which places the group well within the clinical range. Three fifths (61.7%) of participants were underweight at admission into the trial meeting criteria for anorexia nervosa (AN); the remainder met criteria for atypical AN. Depression, Anxiety, and Stress Scale scores fell within the 'severe' range across depression, anxiety and stress (measured by the Depression, Anxiety, and Stress Scale; Lovibond & Lovibond, 1995). Around half of participants (51.6%) reported being prescribed psychotropic medication.

Four fifths of participants (80.3%) had received previous psychological therapy, and the average illness duration was 9.0 years, indicating that this was a chronically unwell group of people. Indeed, compared with other intervention studies with this clinical group, SPEAKS participants started with higher average baseline EDEQ global scores. Furthermore, average illness durations exceeded the expected length for people with 'severe and enduring AN' (Broomfield et al., 2017; Byrne et al., 2017). These and other severity factors such as psychotropic medication use and anxiety/depression symptoms were also greater than other trial participants, including trials conducted for people with 'severe and enduring AN' (Touyz et al., 2013).

Feasibility Findings

The SPEAKS feasibility trial firstly sought to assess the feasibility of SPEAKS as a clinical intervention. It examined *engagement* as indicated by the percentage of people who dropped out through lack of engagement with the therapy. The trial had no clients (0%) who dropped out of therapy. This high level of engagement is particularly striking and significant in a population where drop-out from therapy is reported to be up to 40% (DeJong et al., 2012). Clinical feasibility was addressed by recording numbers of hospitalisations and deaths during the trial. Hospitalisations comprised 2.9% of the sample (within the 2–3% normal range of people attending outpatient therapy in the services recruited from), and there were no deaths.

Therapists largely adhered to the therapy delivery and 87.5% of sessions followed the SPEAKS guidebook. The average number of sessions was 40 and average length was 11 months 1 day, which fell within the expected overall length of therapy (9–12 months).

In order to establish the feasibility of the study methods to inform a future trial, the study also examined eligibility rates (% of people screened who met criteria) and recruitment rates (% of people approached who agreed to take part), which both fell well within expected ranges suggesting that it is possible to recruit to a trial of SPEAKS. Research follow-up rates (research appointments attended) were very high (88.1%), especially for this clinical group, and indicate that participants also engaged well with the research procedures put in place. Furthermore, qualitative analysis of interviews conducted after therapy indicated that most participants found study procedures and measures acceptable. All participants were supportive of a larger trial of SPEAKS.

Acceptability Findings

Following therapy, all participants and therapists were offered post-therapy interviews (Rennick et al., 2024). Semi-structured interviews followed an interview schedule asking questions relating to participant experience of SPEAKS, intervention acceptability, and acceptability of research methods. Interviews were conducted with 16 of the 34 eligible clients and six of the seven eligible therapists. Results of thematic analysis indicated clearly that SPEAKS was considered an acceptable intervention for AN from the perspective of both therapists and clients, who found the intervention afforded new ways to think about and address difficulties. Participants reported finding the techniques which SPEAKS utilises powerful and empowering, although 'chair work' was difficult for some in the first instance. The focus on emotions was broadly welcomed by participants, who identified this as being of importance for creating long-lasting change, whilst therapists welcomed the process-oriented approach. It was concluded that the findings provide strong support for delivery of a larger scale randomised control trial.

Signals of Efficacy

Questionnaires to assess change to a range of clinical factors including eating disorder symptoms (EDEQ global score), anxiety and depression (DASS), and quality of life (Clinical Impairment Assessment [CIA]; Bohn & Fairburn, 2008) were completed via online video platform/telephone at several timepoints including baseline (before beginning therapy) and then every 3 months until 12 months. Body Mass Index (weight in kg/height in metres squared; BMI) for each timepoint was extracted from clinical records.

EDEQ global scores significantly decreased with medium effect from 4.14 pre-therapy (sd = 1.11) to 2.90 post-therapy (sd = 1.74), ($p < 0.000$). For those underweight at the start of therapy ($n = 21$), BMI significantly increased from pre- to post- therapy ($p < 0.001$), with medium effect. Significant pre- to post-therapy reduction of medium to large effect was observed for anxiety ($p < 0.000$), depression ($p < 0.000$) and stress ($p < 0.000$), shifting average score categories from 'severe' at pre-therapy to 'mild' at post-therapy. Quality of life scores (CIA) significantly improved with large effect ($p < 0.000$).

Change Process Research

Change process research enables better understanding of how psychological therapy produces change for the client. It includes, but extends beyond, process outcome designs and pays attention to processes of change within the therapeutic space, and the temporal order in which they occur, affording consideration of both how and why change occurs (Elliott, 2010). SPEAKS includes several hypotheses of change processes argued to be associated with clinical change, and the feasibility trial was an opportunity to test these. Key hypotheses tested were *emotional change* and *change in the 'Self'* (depicted in Figure 3.1) assessed using a range of mixed methodologies.

Utilising the experience of participants and therapists in the feasibility trial, Papastavrou Brooks et al. (under review) explored therapeutic change processes during the SPEAKS intervention described in qualitative interviews. They were conducted with 16 of the 34 eligible clients and six of the seven eligible therapists, following an interview schedule based on the Change Process Interview (Rodgers & Elliott, 2014) and analysed using a reflexive thematic analysis (Braun & Clarke, 2006) by researchers external to the SPEAKS research team to increase validity of findings (alongside analysis of acceptability data described above).

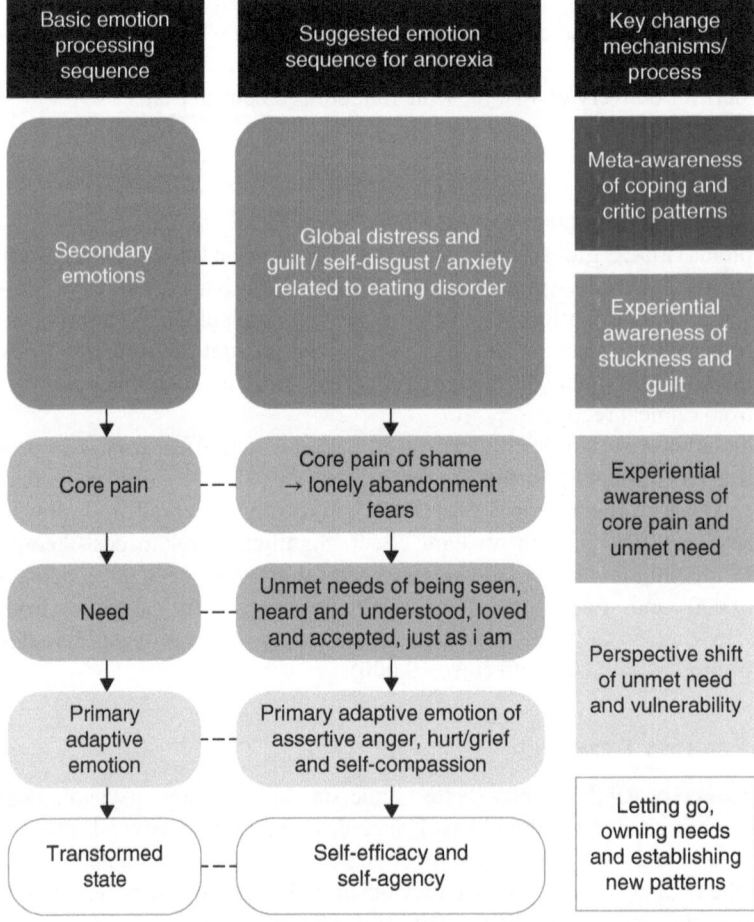

Figure 3.1 Hypothesised emotion change processes and mechanisms of change for each phase

Additional change process research (Malik-Smith et al., in prep) tracked moment-to-moment emotional expression for those with highest 'good' outcomes (weight and ED behaviours both in the 'normal range' at the end of therapy) versus those with most 'poor' outcomes (one or both metrics outside 'normal' range) in video-recorded therapy sessions drawn from three, six, and nine months into therapy (to reflect the key processing phases of therapy: Phases 2/3/4). Sessions were analysed using a tool called the Classification of Affective Meaning States (CAMS) and were conducted by a researcher external to the SPEAKS research team who was blind to both participant group and phase in therapy.

Finally, questionnaires pertaining to emotional change, change in frequency of different 'modes', and qualitative description and pictural change of modes and their interacting relationships were explored (Mountain, 2022). Some key findings from these change process studies are described in what follows.

Emotion Change Processes

Qualitative thematic analysis of post-therapy interviews identified a main theme of emotional change (Papastavrou Brooks et al., 2025), indicative of emotional processing. Client participants reported that prior to receiving SPEAKS they had attempted to hide or suppress emotions, putting them in a box which ran the risk of 'overflowing'. After SPEAKS they were able to tune-in more, acknowledge, listen to, and express how they felt. This was attributed to a range of different mechanisms.

These mechanisms included managing emotion:

I think it's made me be a bit more confident in sitting with negative emotions. (client, female)

Understanding emotion:

One thing I want to add actually, it's not only helped me understand clients, but it's helped me understand myself better ... so I've become much more aware of the different parts of myself and who is at play and what I need. (therapist)

And valuing emotion:

I think I thought to show your emotions was a sign of weakness. Whereas now my view is more, actually, no, sometimes it can be sign of strength to show your vulnerabilities and it takes guts to show your vulnerabilities. So that's a real shift for me. (client, female)

These findings were triangulated by questionnaire data (Mountain, Yim, Startup & Oldershaw, in prep). Beliefs about the unacceptability of emotion (e.g. "I should not let myself give in to 'negative' feelings.") on the Beliefs about Emotions Scale

(Rimes & Chalder, 2010) significantly decreased from pre- to post-therapy with large effect (p < 0.000). Post-therapy scores (mean total = 34.8) were equivalent to that observed in other samples recovered from anorexia (Oldershaw et al., 2012). Furthermore, emotion regulation difficulties significantly reduced with large effect from pre- to post-therapy (p < 0.01), as measured by the Difficulties with Emotion Regulation Scale (Gratz & Roemer, 2004).

The CAMS tool tracked specific emotions expressed during therapy sessions, including which emotion response type they were (secondary, primary maladaptive [core pain], primary adaptive) and temporal patterns, also comparing those with 'good' or 'poor' outcomes from therapy (Malik-Smith et al., in prep). It sought to examine whether the hypothesised emotion change process from secondary emotions to primary maladaptive (core pain) to primary adaptive emotion was observed and whether it related to outcome. There was no significant difference in overall secondary emotion expression between the 'good' and 'poor' outcome groups and no significant difference in overall primary maladaptive emotion, but the good outcome group expressed significantly more primary adaptive emotion than the poor outcome group, with this group difference becoming apparent mid-therapy. Primary maladaptive emotions of shame and lonely abandonment explored separately over time indicated no significant difference between therapy phases for primary maladaptive shame. However, primary maladaptive abandonment fear did significantly reduce for the 'good' outcome group across therapy phases, with less fear expressed in later phases. In contrast, there was no statistical change in abandonment fears for the poor outcome group. This supports the proposed need for and process of resolving core pain in SPEAKS, highlighting emphasis on connecting with lonely abandonment fears (as opposed to just shame) in facilitating change.

Changing the Self

Changing the Self was identified as a second key theme in qualitative interviews post-therapy (Papastavrou Brooks et al., 2025). The changing Self was linked to emotional change; clients were better able to understand and relate to more vulnerable or emotional parts of themselves. Clients and therapists overwhelmingly expressed beliefs that SPEAKS was able to get to the heart of issues and vulnerabilities and that this facilitated understanding of the Self. Initial reluctance to discuss the past was reported by some clients, yet they subsequently found understanding the contribution of past events to their issues enabled identification of underlying behaviours, triggers and core beliefs pertaining to their ED difficulties. Insight into these factors generated a greater sense of control in their current lives, reducing self-criticism and guilt.

> But I really, really do believe with SPEAKS and it really shifting my perspective in terms of getting to the heart of my vulnerability and connecting to my childhood self and where that behaviour all came from and understanding the boundaries I need to put in place for certain people. (client, female)

Most clients reported increased self-confidence, less self-doubt, increased inner strength, feeling "way more comfortable in [their] own skin", and reduction in experiences of shame and guilt as they understood their past better.

I think maybe I'm more confident and, yes, I guess more self-assured … I think it's probably because I feel more deserving, and worthy of the external praise and kind of validation. (client, female)

These findings were triangulated by questionnaire data using the Silencing the Self Scale (Jack & Dill, 1992) which consists of 31 items across four subscales (rated from strongly disagree to strongly agree) and can be seen to reflect the use of coping behaviour pertaining to intimacy: (i) Externalised self-perception (the inclination to judge the Self by external standards); (ii) Care as self-sacrifice (securing attachments by putting needs of others before the Self); (iii) Silencing the Self (inhibiting self-expression to avoid conflict and to preserve relationships); and (iv) Divided Self (presenting an outer compliant self despite the inner self being angry and hostile). Significant reductions in agreement were observed across all four subscales from pre- to post-therapy (all $p < 0.01$), with large effect sizes, supporting qualitative descriptions of changing boundaries and expectations in relationships with others.

In further mixed methods research, client participant formulation maps indicating self-identified parts of self (or schema modes) were analysed alongside scores on a questionnaire to explore frequency of modes, the Schema Mode Inventory for Eating Disorders (SMI, Simpson et al., 2018; rated 0 not present, up to maximum of 5 frequently present) (Mountain, 2022). A key goal of SPEAKS is that the 'Healthy Adult' emerges during therapy. This study found that pre-therapy the Healthy Adult was included on only 58% of formulation maps, most commonly described as "not on the map" or the "furthest part from the [Little Me]". After therapy, the Healthy Adult was on 100% of maps and most commonly described in terms reflecting having 'awareness of the other parts'. A significant increase in endorsement of the frequency of the Healthy Adult on the SMI was found from pre- to post-therapy ($p < 0.05$). Furthermore, before therapy there was no relationship between endorsement of the Healthy Adult and Eating Disorder symptoms and behaviours on the EDEQ, however, after therapy frequency of the Healthy Adult significantly predicted post-therapy eating disorder thoughts and behaviours, with a more frequently present Healthy Adult linked to reduced eating disorder thoughts and behaviours ($p < 0.001$).

Testing SPEAKS: Conclusion

The SPEAKS intervention was developed from evidential work and informed by the theoretical underpinnings of Emotion Focused Therapy and Schema Therapy. The feasibility study outcomes and change process outcomes point to the justification and desirability of the next step of conducting a Randomised Control Trial in order to further evaluate the effectiveness of the therapy. The emphasis on emotional change processes found in the data aligns with hypothesised mechanisms of change in the SPEAKS model and how changes in eating disorder outcomes can be facilitated in therapy. They mirror qualitative SPEAKS intervention development work which highlighted the need to 'see emotions differently' and connect with emotions and self as core processes for recovery and growth (Drinkwater et al., 2022).

References

Bohn, K., & Fairburn, C. G. (2008). The clinical impairment assessment questionnaire (CIA). In C. G. Fairburn (Ed.) *Cognitive behavioral therapy for eating disorders*, (315–317). Guilford Press.

Braun, V., & Clarke, V. (2006). Using thematic analysis in psychology. *Qualitative Research in Psychology*, *3*(2), 77–101.

Brooks, C. P., Rennick, A., Basra, R. S., Lavender, T., Startup, H., & Oldershaw, A. (2025). "It's OK for Me to Cry": Client and Therapist Perspectives on Change Processes in SPEAKS Therapy for Anorexia Nervosa. *Journal of clinical psychology*, 10.1002/jclp.23769. Advance online publication. https://doi.org/10.1002/jclp.23769

Broomfield, C., Stedal, K., Touyz, S., & Rhodes, P. (2017). Labeling and defining severe and enduring anorexia nervosa: A systematic review and critical analysis. *International Journal of Eating Disorders*, *50*(6), 611–623.

Byrne, S., Wade, T., Hay, P., Touyz, S., Fairburn, C., Treasure, J., Schmidt, U., McIntosh, V., Allen, K., & Fursland, A. (2017). A randomised controlled trial of three psychological treatments for anorexia nervosa. *Psychological Medicine*, *47*(16), 2823–2833.

DeJong, H., Broadbent, H., & Schmidt, U. (2012). A systematic review of dropout from treatment in outpatients with anorexia nervosa. *International Journal of Eating Disorders*, *45*(5), 635–647.

Drinkwater, D., Holttum, S., Lavender, T., Startup, H., & Oldershaw, A. (2022). Seeing through the façade of anorexia: A grounded theory of emotional change processes associated with recovery from anorexia nervosa. *Frontiers in Psychiatry*, *13*, 1316.

Elliott, R. (2010). Psychotherapy change process research: Realizing the promise. *Psychotherapy Research*, *20*(2), 123–135.

Fairburn, C. G., & Beglin, S. J. (2008). Eating disorder examination questionnaire. *Cognitive Behavior Therapy and Eating Disorders*, *309*, 313.

Gratz, K. L., & Roemer, L. (2004). Multidimensional assessment of emotion regulation and dysregulation: Development, factor structure, and initial validation of the difficulties in emotion regulation scale. *Journal of Psychopathology and Behavioral Assessment*, *26*, 41–54.

Jack, D. C., & Dill, D. (1992). The Silencing the Self Scale: Schemas of intimacy associated with depression in women. *Psychology of Women Quarterly*, *16*(1), 97–106.

Lovibond, P. F., & Lovibond, S. H. (1995). The structure of negative emotional states: Comparison of the Depression Anxiety Stress Scales (DASS) with the Beck Depression and Anxiety Inventories. *Behaviour Research and Therapy*, *33*(3), 335–343.

Malik-Smith, S., Papastavrou Brooks., C., Callanan, M., Pascual-Leone, A. & Oldershaw, A. (in prep). The process of emotion change associated with recovery from anorexia nervosa.

Mountain, L. (2022). *Formulation and anorexia nervosa.* Canterbury Christ Church University (United Kingdom).

Mountain, L., Yim, V., Startup, H. & Oldershaw, A. (in prep). Integration of the 'Healthy Adult' and the 'Little Self' in recovery from anorexia nervosa.

Oldershaw, A., Basra, R. S., Lavender, T., & Startup, H. (2024). Specialist Psychotherapy with Emotion for Anorexia in Kent and Sussex: An intervention development and non-randomised single arm feasibility trial. *European Eating Disorders Review, 32*(2), 215–229.

Oldershaw, A., DeJong, H., Hambrook, D., Broadbent, H., Tchanturia, K., Treasure, J., & Schmidt, U. (2012). Emotional processing following recovery from anorexia nervosa. *European Eating Disorders Review, 20*(6), 502–509.

Rennick, A., Papastavrou Brooks, C., Singh Basra, R., Startup, H., Lavender, T., & Oldershaw, A. (2024). Acceptability of Specialist Psychotherapy with Emotion for Anorexia in Kent and Sussex (SPEAKS): A novel intervention for anorexia nervosa. *International Journal of Eating Disorders, 57*(3), 611–623.

Rimes, K. A., & Chalder, T. (2010). The Beliefs about Emotions Scale: Validity, reliability and sensitivity to change. *Journal of psychosomatic research, 68*(3), 285–292.

Rodgers, B., & Elliott, R. (2014). Qualitative methods in psychotherapy outcome research. In O. C. G. Gelo, A. Pritz, & B. Rieken (Eds.), *Psychotherapy research: Foundations, process, and outcome* (pp. 559–578). Springer.

Simpson, S. G., Pietrabissa, G., Rossi, A., Seychell, T., Manzoni, G. M., Munro, C., Nesci, J. B., & Castelnuovo, G. (2018). Factorial structure and preliminary validation of the Schema Mode Inventory for Eating Disorders (SMI-ED). *Frontiers in Psychology, 9*, 600.

Touyz, S., Le Grange, D., Lacey, H., Hay, P., Smith, R., Maguire, S., Bamford, B., Pike, K. M., & Crosby, R. D. (2013). Treating severe and enduring anorexia nervosa: A randomized controlled trial. *Psychological Medicine, 43*(12), 2501–2511.

Section II

Section II

Chapter 4

SPEAKS Therapy Overview

Introduction to the Five SPEAKS phases

The Specialist Psychotherapy with Emotion for Anorexia in Kent and Sussex (SPEAKS) process-based model is divided into five treatment phases (see Figure 4.1): Engagement & Formulation – Building a narrative (Phase 1), Seeing through and Moving past the Façade of Anorexia (Phase 2), Deepening to Core Pain (Phase 3), Resolving Core Pain (Phase 4), and Consolidating the 'Real Me' (Phase 5).

Each treatment phase has its own goals with associated change processes facilitated by therapeutic 'tasks'. Formulation via the use of a 'mode map' sets out 'parts of the self' (Jacob & Arntz, 2013) – including coping modes such as those associated with secondary emotions, alongside the core pain of the Little Self, the Eating Disorder Part (EDP), the Inner Critic – and highlights relationships between them. This formulation occurs early in therapy during Phase 1, indicating facilitators and blocks to the SPEAKS process of emotion change for a particular client. Within session 'markers' indicate a client's 'live' processes and point to the use of a specific task to work with what is present in each session (Elliott & Greenberg, 2007). The sequential model of emotion processing and change outlined in Chapter 2 maps onto the treatment phases (see Figure 4.2). This change process is encased in a broader range of work from 'mode mapping' and relationship building topping the therapy in Phase 1 to the consolidation of emotional, behavioural and cognitive change (the 'Real Me') characteristic of Phase 5.

The phases are considered to be 'soft', and it is recognised that clients will move backwards and forwards through them. The EDP, coping modes and blocks to emotional change continue to be triggered throughout therapy before they are sufficiently resolved. Indeed, this two-steps forward, one-step back progress through therapy is argued to a be valuable aspect of the therapeutic process and observed to be associated with better outcomes (Pascual-Leone, 2018).

DOI: 10.4324/9781003468349-6

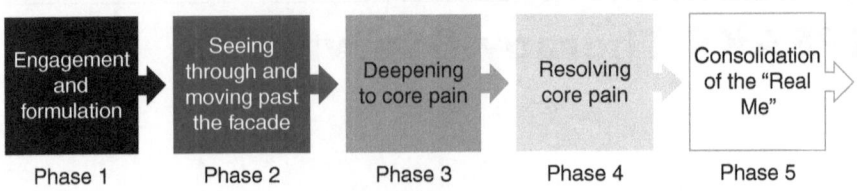

Figure 4.1 The five phases of SPEAKS therapy

Phase 1: Engagement & Formulation – Building a Narrative

Phase 1 (Engagement & Formulation) establishes the groundwork for therapy with key consideration to building a warm, empathic, genuinely caring, and safe therapeutic relationship, central to change. Establishing this relationship includes empathic responding techniques (Greenberg, 2014) and the use of 'limited reparenting' (Gülüm & Soygüt, 2022). This demonstration of a validating, strongly empathic, relationship offers the start of a 'corrective emotional experience' and is integral to the emotion change process.

During Phase 1, therapist and client begin to construct a narrative of anorexia, how it developed over time, and how it helps them (e.g. for emotion regulation; to protect/guard). It is useful to begin, even in the first session, by helping the client to explore and symbolise anorexia and the EDP as well as associated emotions. Understanding and empathy for anorexia as a protector should be expressed by the therapist.

The therapist attunes to expression of emotion and other parts of self as they arise, noting and reflecting these back to the client when revealed within their narrative. Through a process of reflecting this back to the client in the moment, therapist and client will ultimately collaboratively develop a 'whole self' mode map formulation during Phase 1. From the outset, consideration should be given to monitoring risk and exploring the possibility of, and current limits to, behavioural change with regard to food and health.

A summary of Phase 1 is displayed in Table 4.1, and a full description, including of associated tasks and mechanisms of change, is provided in Chapter 5.

Signs Phase 1 Is Moving towards Phase 2

Phase 1 is moving towards Phase 2 when the client has an outline formulation and is ready to consider working with emotion processes and/or their parts of self. The therapeutic relationship should have deepened to establish a sufficiently safe bond to begin to approach emotion more meaningfully. Note that at this stage the client may still be conflicted as to the degree to which they want to move on from

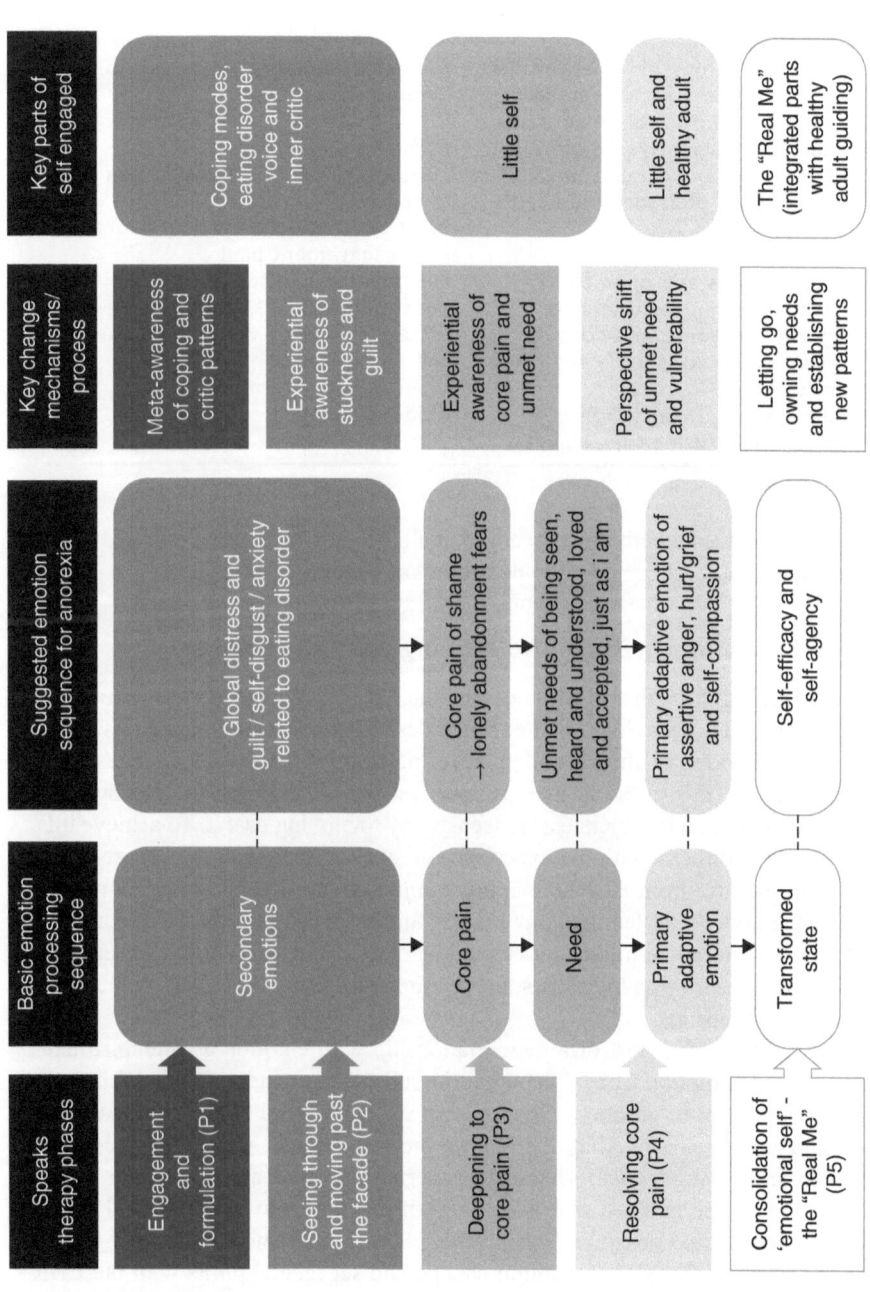

Figure 4.2 SPEAKS therapy flow and map to phases

Table 4.1 Summary of Phase 1 Goals and Tasks

Phase 1 Goals	Suggested Tasks
(1) Building an empathic relationship to create safety for vulnerability and initial emotional expression	• Empathic attunement, validation and 'limited reparenting'
(2) Exploring a narrative of anorexia, its meaning, and establishing management of associated health risks	• Formulation and case conceptualisation: Anorexia as a part of self (EDP) • Psychoeducation on eating disorders & risk management plan
(3) Being curious and open to a client's current experiencing, their inner world, and core relationships to identify their key 'parts of self'/modes	• Formulation and case conceptulisation: Understanding & increasing meta-awareness of parts of self
(4) Representing formulation (drawing out/using toys/objects)	• Mode mapping

anorexia, or indeed whether they want to at all. Moving to Phase 2 requires only a willingness to at least consider the possibility of change.

Phase 2: Seeing through and Moving past the Façade

Phase 2 (Seeing through and Moving past the Façade) aims to further reduce eating disorder (ED) behaviours and enhance desire for and belief in the possibility of change. Working at the secondary level of emotion and coping modes, as is characteristic of this phase in therapy, can feel like a 'stuck place'. Recognising and engaging with this 'stuckness' is seen as key to moving past it. To achieve this, Phase 2 works directly with the experience of stuckness. It aims to support clients to further decentre from EDP, unpicking its motivations, but crucially connecting these to the underlying feelings it provokes, and associated needs. This represents a shift from a more 'cognitive' understanding of the EDP that will have been characteristic of Phase 1 and highlights the emotional impact of the EDP on the client and their relationships.

Phase 2 begins the start of a new relationship with emotion as therapist takes on the role of 'Emotion Coach' in supporting clients to connect with the felt sense and symbolisation of emotion. Clients often express global distress, self-disgust, guilt, and anxiety provoked by the EDP in the first instance (reflecting secondary emotions and coping modes). Using chair work to facilitate a dialogue, the 'noise' of the EDP can be reduced and 'softening' of this part into a less critical stance can even begin to be possible. This affords clients some emotional and cognitive space to consider further behavioural change and set related limits with the EDP. It also opens up access to subsequent emotional work when a 'broader critic' is revealed, who articulates fundamental characterological flaws provoking core pain.

Table 4.2 Summary of Phase 2 Goals and Tasks

Phase 2 Goals	Suggested Tasks
(1) Working with 'stuckness' to better understand the impact and costs of this, linking to current emotion and need	• Focusing on stuckness • Chair work with future selves
(2) Changing relationships with emotion and learning to connect with emotion	• Emotion coaching • Accessing unclear feelings
(3) Exploring the relationship with the EDP and linking this to emotion and need	• Chair work with the EDP
(4) Deepening to the broader critic focused on fundamental flaws	• Chair work with the EDP moving into chair work with the broader Critic (see Phase 3 for elaboration on progressing this work)
(5) Reducing the impact of coping modes as blocks to emotion process work	• Chair work with coping modes (see Phase 3 for elaboration on progressing this work)

Shame about the Self (worthlessness) and of having emotions and needs are usually encountered here. This connection is further elaborated and deepened in Phase 3.

In short, this phase helps clients to begin to see past the 'façade' of the EDP as a protector and a necessary part of their lives, shifting intransigent 'stuckness'. It opens up new possibilities in the client's relationship with and connection to emotion, from feared and avoided to important and worth considering. Table 4.2 summarises Phase 2, and a full description of this phase is provided in Chapter 6.

Signs Phase 2 Is Moving towards Phase 3

Phase 2 moves towards Phase 3 when a client is no longer paralysed in stuckness. There may have been some 'softening' of the EDP, but this can still be tentative until later in therapy. The work with the EDP has 'deepened' to reveal a broader critic, which can be worked with in Phase 3, and on some level, the client has been able to access or more readily recognise the 'Little Self'; this is likely to reflect a move from secondary emotions of global distress/helplessness (reflective of coping modes) to core pain of shame of the Self and of having needs. A goal is set for Phase 3 to further loosen blocks and to work with the broader critic, such that a gradually deeper and authentic connection with emotions can be achieved.

Phase 3: Deepening to Core Pain

Across SPEAKS, the therapist sensitively supports the client using tasks and techniques to facilitate a sequence of emotional processing (Pascual-Leone, 2018).

Once the work in Phase 2 has deepened to involve some experience of core pain (likely shame about the self and of having emotions and needs), the work has entered Phase 3. The aim of Phase 3 is to further deepen this emotional experience and to '*Follow the Pain*'.

Working with the EDP in Phase 2 is seen as a means to reveal and connect with an underlying 'broader critic' whose origins and functions can be explored. This enables connection to and work with core pain and associated unmet needs. Expression of and connection with painful emotion and internalised messages associated with shame (e.g. "You do not deserve good things; you are too broken/ defective") that can be furthered into lonely abandonment feelings and related messages ("So if you show yourself to others they will reject you. You are unworthy of love and connection and are completely alone in life") gives way to the Little Self's connection with and expression of the needs aligned with these core painful feelings: "I needed to be heard/seen, to know I was worth something in your eyes, to feel your love and closeness." This core pain and unmet need are linked to episodic memories, grounding them within the developmental relationships in which they emerged. Phase 4 subsequently builds on this connection to transform stuck old emotional and relational patterns and facilitate the emergence of the 'Healthy Adult' (Oldershaw & Startup, 2020).

It is recognised that clients will move backwards and forwards between phases, as clients approach and retreat from core painful feelings. Also noted is that tolerance for emotion work will vary and may need to be moderated or approached at different rates depending upon the client, with close attention paid to emotion regulation requirements and capacity. Clients will access emotional processing in different ways, with some clients accessing emotion more overtly, deeply, or experientially than others. Furthermore, blocks to accessing emotions in the form of coping modes will likely arise. Here therapist attunement is a crucial guide, and clinicians are sensitive and flexible, working alongside the client's processing style to move between tasks with a more emotional, cognitive, or behavioural basis, whilst maintaining their therapeutic stance of empathy and 'limited reparenting'. Table 4.3 summarises Phase 3, and a full description is provided in Chapter 7.

Signs Phase 3 Is Moving towards Phase 4

Simply put, Phase 3 moves into Phase 4 when core pain has been experienced and elaborated. Of note is that Phase 3 flows into Phase 4 seamlessly in a process of emotion transformation with some tasks (e.g. chair work with the broader Critic; float back) straddling both phases. Furthermore, there will be considerable movement back and forth between these phases, and even back to Phase 2. They are merely separated for the purposes of explanation of process and to extrapolate the different issues encountered with each part of the process.

Table 4.3 Summary of Phase 3 Goals and Tasks

Phase 3 Goals	Suggested Tasks
(1) Deepening to a connection with core pain	• Chair work with the 'broader' Inner Critic • Float back task • Empathic responding and attunement
(2) Linking core pain with unmet developmental need and relationships as well as to external and internal ways of relating (links to narrative and/or formulation)	• Chair work with the 'broader' Inner Critic • Float back task • Make links to mode map
(3) Continuing work to remove blocks to emotion processing (e.g. by bypassing coping modes)	• Chair work with coping modes
(4) Optimising emotion regulation	• Taught tasks for self-soothing, e.g. safe bubble and/or safe place • Audio flash cards

Phase 4: Resolving Core Pain

Once a connection with the core pain of the Little Self has been achieved, the client is supported to transform and resolve that core pain in a process of 'changing emotion with emotion' achieved via underlying mechanisms of memory reconsolidation and the corrective emotional experience (Greenberg et al., 2024). The expression of needs associated with core pain (especially those associated with feelings of lonely abandonment/attachment fears) gives way to concurrent primary adaptive emotions of grief and sadness followed by assertive/protective anger that these needs could not be fully met in early developmental relationships. From here other adaptive emotions such as self-compassion arise. These newly emerging emotions, and in particular their associated action tendencies, are core features of the Healthy Adult.

The intrapersonal experience of self-compassion (as opposed to self-soothing) is more explicitly considered here. For this particular client group, who demonstrate such strong coping modes of compliant surrenderer and detached protectors, these blocks to self-compassion must be at least partly overcome before the client can truly begin to believe and 'feel' that they might deserve compassion. Connecting with primary adaptive emotions further supports this facilitation. Indeed, self-compassion is directed from the Healthy Adult; therefore, this part of self must be at least emerging in order for compassion to be authentically expressed in a way that connects in a 'felt sense'. Such explicit, connecting self-validation further strengthens the Healthy Adult and consolidates the basis for new ways of

Table 4.4 Summary of Phase 4 Goals and Tasks

Phase 4 Goals	Suggested Tasks
(1) Emotion transformation (including memory reconsolidation and corrective emotional experience)	• Float back with imagery rescripting • Empty chair 'unfinished business' task • Revisiting tasks described in Phase 3, such as chair work with the broader Inner Critic now that adaptive emotion is more accessible and the Healthy Adult more available.
(2) Building self-compassion	• Chair work (with the Little Self) for self-compassion

navigating the Self, relationships and the world. Table 4.4 summarises Phase 4, and Chapter 8 provides a full description of the phase and associated tasks.

Signs Phase 4 Is Moving towards Phase 5

Phase 4 is moving towards Phase 5 when primary adaptive emotion has been accessed and the Healthy Adult who demonstrates assertive/protective anger and self-compassion has begun to more consistently emerge. This part may still be tentative, but there is a shift in the client's self-organisation that is the foundation for the 'Real Me'.

Phase 5: The 'Real Me'

By Phase 5, the client has arrived at and worked to transform their core pain. By experiencing and expressing adaptive emotions, the Self is strengthened and feels more motivated to break free from limiting avoidant processes (Elliott et al., 2016). Clients are beginning to connect transformed emotional experience to new and alternative intra- and interpersonal ways of responding that reflect a more resilient and integrated sense of self. Indeed, it is argued that only once a cohesive and stable sense of self has emerged that people with AN can successfully process and manage situations inherent to recovery, such as gaining weight (Croce et al., 2024).

This phase involves supporting further emergence of and consolidation of the 'Real Me'. This can include encouraging, testing, and prizing of new Healthy Adult ways of being in the world. In addition, recovery is suggested to require a stage of 'letting go of AN' (Amianto et al., 2016). In Phase 5, Chair work with the EDP is revisited to consolidate the Healthy Adult ways of responding and adaptive emotional experience. This also highlights shifts in intrapersonal relationships, as well as pointing to any further work that might need to be considered before ending. It importantly considers approaching and working with the grief and loss of the ED and shifts in the view of this part.

Table 4.5 Summary of Phase 5 Goals and Tasks

Phase 5 Goals	Suggested Tasks
(1) Greater integration of the parts of self and stronger expression of the Healthy Adult exploring getting needs met in healthy and adaptive ways	• Exploration of desired changes and behavioural experiments led by the Healthy Adult
(2) Grieving loss and letting go	• Chair work task with the EDP to process letting go • Revisiting self-compassion chair work
(3) Reviewing progress made and any future changes the client wants to work towards	• Remapping the mode map visually and in written description
(4) Processing therapeutic endings	• Ending letters • Transitional objects

Phase 5 includes the ending of therapy. Central to this is reviewing the work done (e.g. visual and written remapping of the mode map) as well as processing the end of the relationship (e.g. in ending letters). From the therapist's point of view, ending letters are not a clinical letter per se, but one of the last ways the therapist can connect with their client from one human being to another via their own Healthy Adult as they reflect on their own emotional processes and express their authentic adaptive primary feelings in response to the ending.

There is continuation of the emotion transformation process in the ending of the corrective emotional experience and transitional objects can be given as a reminder of the time spent together and of key shifts made, as appropriate. Client and therapist may agree to meet less often at this point, gradually tapering the frequency of sessions. On average SPEAKS therapy for people with anorexia lasts 40 sessions (Oldershaw et al., 2024). Table 4.5 summarises Phase 5, and Chapter 9 provides a full description.

SPEAKS Therapy Sessions in Practice

The focus and course of the SPEAKS intervention, as a whole and within each specific session, is subject to therapist judgement and individual client needs, guided by therapist attunement. The phases of SPEAKS are 'soft' and it is expected and welcomed that clients will move backwards and forwards across phases/tasks. Therapists are listening for 'markers' present in client's narratives as they engage with each session to give an indication of client processes and emotions engaged. These 'markers' highlight different sorts of problematic processing and indicate the usefulness of specific tasks in that moment to work with the client's current experiential process (Elliott & Greenberg, 2007). As a rough guide, we provide some indication of how individual sessions and the pattern of sessions during the overall therapy may look.

Active Task-based Sessions

A task-focused session means one in which a piece of chair work or active experiential intervention is selected and worked with. Each active task-focused therapy session in SPEAKS follows a roughly similar outline as follows.

Part 1 – Watch and Wait for a Session Focus

During the first part of the session therapist invites the client to bring their narrative from the past week. Therapists can invite clients to share with them in their usual way or by asking clients if there is something that they would like to focus on this week. Therapists are responding with empathic attunement and listening for a marker (an indication of problematic processing early in a session pointing to a specific task as beneficial). It may be that there is more than one marker arising in what a client brings. Sometimes it can help to ask the client what they would like to focus on this week; however it is a therapist's aim to try to differentiate which is the marker with the most salient emotion. This section may take 10–15 minutes or may be much shorter if the marker is clear or if therapist and client collaboratively bookmarked a focus in the previous session that still feels relevant and important.

Part 2 – Task

The middle part of the session will be devoted to task completion. In the early stages of therapy it is likely that one task will be completed per session. As therapy progresses, one task may naturally lead into another, such as an 'unfinished business' task moving into self-compassion chair work.

Part 3 – Debrief

For the final ten minutes or so of the session, a client moves out of the task and back into conversation directly with the therapist. This is an opportunity to reflect on the task, what was experienced, and to make sense of it. It may be (especially early in therapy) that the client does not move past the first few steps of a task. This does not mean the task has failed, it will always shed light on important aspects of the client's process and blocks or facilitators of that. It is important not to leave the client in a vulnerable state that is too raw (exposed Little Self) as they leave the therapy room and some regulation work may be needed. The therapist will gain their client's perspective and share what they observed as important or meaningful. In this part of the session therapist and client can draw links back to the formulation and mode map as appropriate. Here it may also be appropriate to include some psy-choeducation (e.g. around the nature of weight gain or around emotion processing) and instilling hope as the session is coming to an end, using a 'reparenting' stance as appropriate. At the end/after the session it may also be helpful to provide visual or written summaries of key aspects of what has been discussed for neurodivergent people (Mason et al., 2023).

Sessions without Experiential Tasks

Sometimes therapists feel they have to do a chair work or imagery task every session, but not every session will revolve around an experiential task. It is the therapist's judgement and their responsiveness to markers that indicates whether a task is appropriate or not, and there is no recommended pattern. It may be that, for a couple of weeks, there are active emotional deepening tasks and then no experiential tasks for a couple of weeks.

Indicators that an (emotional deepening) task should not be used might be that:

- The client accessed very deep emotion during the previous active task session and is in a vulnerable space the following week, thus they may need a more supportive reparenting and empathic session, involving a soothing task or containment.
- The client revealed something during an active task the previous week which needs some specific attention in narrative retelling.
- The active task revealed a complex number of threads which require additional information and/or detailed linking back to the formulation.
- Attention needs to be given to other practical clinical demands taking priority, including risk assessment or physical health.
- For neurodivergent people, consideration given to 'energy accounting' (weighing up energy withdrawals and deposits to both guard and replenish them; Attwood, 2020) may mean pacing therapy more slowly and allowing more recovery from deeply emotional sessions, without losing momentum.

How to Use This Guidebook

The remainder of this book is given over to what is essentially a manual for SPEAKS therapy, guiding therapists through the five phases and delivery of each task. It is important to remember that although we outline an overall therapy trajectory, clients will move backwards and forwards between phases. Thus, we describe this book as a guidebook to reflect that it is not rigid in its delivery and is reliant upon therapist skill and attunement to moment-to-moment client experience. SPEAKS should be delivered by trained therapists. Additional training in one or more emotion and/or relational therapeutic model(s) and/or for their clinical supervisor to be Emotion Focused Therapy or Schema Therapy trained is beneficial.

SPEAKS training for therapists is also available to obtain experiential, supervised skills practice of SPEAKS tasks.

Of note is that eating disorders are over-represented in neurodivergent populations (Cobbaert & Rose, 2023) and neurodivergent people do less well from therapy modalities currently available for eating disorders (Leppanen et al., 2022). As such, working therapeutically with people with eating disorders means that we are commonly also working with neurodivergent people. This should be acknowledged, and it is important to consider effective ways to adapt what we offer to meet a range of needs. Throughout this guidebook we provide reflections on and suggested adaptations of tasks and their instructions for working with neurodivergent clients. Here we use identity-first language to reflect the preference of most autistic and other neurodivergent people. This stems from a desire to reframe autism as core to sense of self and identity and which is to be embraced, rather than perceiving it as a 'disorder' to be cured (Cobbaert & Rose, 2023). Although identity-first language is the preference of the majority in the autistic community, it is recommended to discuss this openly with clients as some may still prefer person-first language (e.g. person with autism).

Table 4.6 Overview of Clara's Presentation to Therapy

Clara – This Guidebook's SPEAKS Therapy Client
Clara is a 32-year-old female. She lives with her fiancé and their dog in a town in south-east England. She works in pressurised job in a city office as a management consultant. Clara grew up living with her mum, dad, and two brothers and is the middle child. Her mum and dad both worked full-time and the children often went to after-school care. Clara describes her mum as a "Workaholic" and that life was always on overdrive. Her dad was "larger than life". Life revolved around her brothers' sporting fixtures and her mum and dad's social life. Clara described a lot of having to "fit in" with what others wanted and needed and always feeling different to everyone else.
Clara currently presents with a diagnosis of anorexia nervosa. Her BMI is 17.3. Her eating disorder behaviours are food restriction and excessive exercise. There is no binging, purging by vomiting, or self-harm. She came to therapy due to work burnout and feeling mentally exhausted. She is aware that anorexia has been ticking around in the background for as long as she can remember, and she had some therapy previously aged 14, but the work situation has highlighted her need for support. As an adult, Clara has been diagnosed with attention deficit hyperactivity disorder (ADHD) and recognises this drives her towards trying to control and hyper-organise at work to compensate for difficulties in this area, which feeds her sense of inadequacy and her fear of failure.
Clara is ambivalent about change and spoke about how the eating disorder helps her to achieve more and gives her a buzz. She presents with everything is "fine" and her main motivation to come to therapy was around improving her work situation and to please others. Her current intrinsic motivation for change pertaining to eating and exercise is low.

Throughout the guidebook we will use a case example to illustrate how therapy might progress. Our client, Clara, and her therapist will appear through the task descriptions. We introduce Clara as she presented to therapy in Table 4.6. Clara is a fictitious client, yet one born out of our collective therapeutic exerience of working with this client group and chosen to highlight a realistic SPEAKS client. All resources presented as relating to Clara have been developed specifically for this guidebook and are not actual client accounts/resources. Our aim in drawing upon one clinical presentation is so the reader can follow the character's journey and ensuing therapeutic processes as responded to through SPEAKS. Of course, a SPEAKS therapeutic journey will look very different depending on the client and even Clara's journey would have been more detailed and nuanced than it is possible to express here.

References

Amianto, F., Northoff, G., Abbate Daga, G., Fassino, S., & Tasca, G. A. (2016). Is anorexia nervosa a disorder of the self? A psychological approach. *Frontiers in psychology, 7*, 186132.

Attwood, T. (2020). Working with individuals on the spectrum. In R. Bedard & L. Hecker (Eds.), *A spectrum of solutions for clients with autism* (pp. 3–13). Routledge.

Cobbaert, L., & Rose, A. (2023). *Eating disorders and neurodivergence: A stepped care approach.* Eating Disorders Neurodiversity Australia; National Eating Disorders Collaboration (NEDC).

Croce, S. R., Malcolm, A. C., Ralph-Nearman, C., & Phillipou, A. (2024). The role of identity in anorexia nervosa: a narrative review. *New Ideas in Psychology, 72*, 101060.

Elliott, R., & Greenberg, L. S. (2007). The essence of process-experiential/emotion-focused therapy. *American Journal of Psychotherapy, 61*(3), 241–254.

Elliott, R., & Shahar, B. (2019). Emotion-focused therapy for social anxiety. In L. S. Greenberg & R. N. Goldman (Eds.), *Clinical handbook of emotion-focused therapy* (pp. 337–360). American Psychological Association.

Greenberg, L. (2014). The therapeutic relationship in emotion-focused therapy. *Psychotherapy, 51*(3), 350.

Greenberg, L., Pascual-Leone, J., & Johnson, J. (2024). Schematic processing and emotional change: Implications for treatment. *New Ideas in Psychology, 73*, 101075.

Gülüm, İ. V., & Soygüt, G. (2022). Limited reparenting as a corrective emotional experience in schema therapy: A preliminary task analysis. *Psychotherapy Research, 32*(2), 263–276.

Jacob, G. A., & Arntz, A. (2013). Schema therapy for personality disorders—A review. *International Journal of Cognitive Therapy, 6*(2), 171–185.

Leppanen, J., Sedgewick, F., Halls, D., & Tchanturia, K. (2022). Autism and anorexia nervosa: longitudinal prediction of eating disorder outcomes. *Frontiers in Psychiatry, 13*, 985867.

Mason, D., Acland, J., Stark, E., Happé, F., & Spain, D. (2023). Compassion-focused therapy with autistic adults. *Frontiers in Psychology, 14*, 1267968.

Oldershaw, A., Basra, R. S., Lavender, T., & Startup, H. (2024). Specialist Psychotherapy with Emotion for Anorexia in Kent and Sussex: An intervention development and non-randomised single arm feasibility trial. *European Eating Disorders Review*, *32*(2), 215–229.

Oldershaw, A., & Startup, H. (2020). Building the healthy adult in eating disorders: A schema mode and emotion-focused therapy approach for anorexia nervosa. In G. Heath & H. Startup (Eds.), *Creative methods in schema therapy* (pp. 287–300). Routledge.

Pascual-Leone, A. (2018). How clients "change emotion with emotion": A programme of research on emotional processing. *Psychotherapy Research*, *28*(2), 165–182.

Phase 1

Engagement and Formulation

Chapter 5 outlines core processes involved in Phase 1 of SPEAKS. It starts by discussing the *therapeutic relationship*, seen as establishing the groundwork for therapy. It explains the need for *establishing goals*, including pertaining to early eating disorder (ED) change and risk management. A key aspect of Phase 1 explicated in this chapter is the process of constructing a narrative of anorexia nervosa (AN) and of the parts of self, leading to collaboratively developing a 'whole self' mode map which reflects the *case conceptualisation and formulation*.

The Therapeutic Relationship: The First Task

The psychotherapeutic relationship, also known as the working alliance, is one of the most important and emphasised vehicles for change across psychotherapy models, associated with clinical outcomes (Baier et al., 2020). It holds a central role in both Emotion Focused Therapy (EFT) and Schema Therapy (ST), and is equally fundamental in Specialist Psychotherapy with Emotion for Anorexia in Kent and Sussex (SPEAKS). A therapist who is genuinely empathic, accepting, validating, compassionate, and prizing offers potential for a 'corrective emotional experience' and client healing and growth.

Facilitating a strong working alliance of this nature firstly depends upon therapists being sufficiently empathically attuned to their clients so as to be effective and responsive to their current process and inner emotional world. Therapists open themselves up to their client's experiencing and meet them in it, with warmth, genuineness, and presence. Therapists need good awareness of their own schemas and core pain to be mindful of the 'schema chemistry' that will inevitably arise. This is critical in order to be effectively present and attuned (Roediger & Archonti, 2019). Secondly, they must be able to establish a strong and collaborative working alliance, such that therapist and client explore and facilitate change together as a joint endeavour. Thirdly, they must bring this therapeutic presence and attunement in the delivery of therapeutic techniques and tasks, i.e. a safe therapeutic relationship, promoting emotional co-regulation, in which clients feel secure enough to engage with painful emotions and complete therapeutic tasks. Without this, tasks become ineffective and even harmful. This therapist stance reflects a therapy which

DOI: 10.4324/9781003468349-7

seeks to ecompass "islands of work in an ocean of empathy" (Greenberg, 2017, p. 10).

In this section, we discuss fundamental aspects of establishing and developing the therapeutic relationship specifically focusing on the concepts of *empathic attunement and therapist presence* and *limited reparenting*. We go on to discuss the *therapeutic relationship when working with neurodivergent clients*.

Empathic Attunement and Therapist Presence

Since Freud (1912) first described the phenomenon of transference (cited in Bourdin, 2023), the value of using our experience of clients as a means for understanding within the therapy process has been emphasised by prominent psychotherapists and analysts, such as Winnicott (1960), Kohut (1977), Bowlby (1979) & Rogers (1975). Whilst transference holds the therapist as representative of previous 'old' attachment objects in the client's life, a stance of empathic attunement seeks to help the client experience the therapist as a 'new' and healthier object to be internalised, thereby affording a different opportunity to experience the attachment process in more beneficial ways. Kohut (1977), in his 'self psychology' approach, argues that the task of therapist is to provide a client with a 'corrective emotional experience' via empathy and attunement, with the therapist serving multiple 'self-object' functions, similar to those required of an early caregiver to gratify early unmet needs (Banai et al., 2005). The internalisation of multiple empathic interactions with a therapist, thus can lead to more adaptive modes of thinking, feeling, behaving, and the development of improved self-soothing and emotion regulation capacity. It is the basis for a corrective emotional experience; feeling accepted and emotionally understood in the warmth of the therapist's presence, a client can become more accepting and less self-critical or judgemental. In SPEAKS this affords not only healing of the Little Self, but also the internalisation of new healthy 'objects' supporting the emergence and growth of the Healthy Adult.

In practice, empathic attunement is a moment-by-moment attunement of the therapist to client affect – "keeping one's finger on the client's emotional pulse" (Greenberg, 2021, p. 16). The therapist follows the client experience with empathy, acceptance, and curiosity, tentatively reflecting back understandings of the client's bodily sensations, feelings, meanings, and needs, seeking to fully 'land on' their experience. Therapist empathic attunement, prizing, authenticity, transparency, and collaboration are all primarily communicated through the therapist's manner of being with the client, their presence. Presence is authentically expressed via therapist's tracking body language and non-verbal communication, such as through eye contact and tone of voice. Empathic attunement and therapist presence is thus not a passive experience but one in which the therapist seeks to receive the client and to open themselves up to what their client is bringing in order to understand and usefully respond (Geller & Greenberg, 2023). This level of engagement by the therapist requires them to be present and free of distractions, in touch with their own inner experiences, and self-aware. At this stage in SPEAKS therapy holding an empathically attuned presence is the key focus. Using empathy and ways of empathically responding to guide and deepen client process is further discussed in Phase 2 (Chapter 6).

'Limited Reparenting'

Encompassing and building on the stance of empathic attunement and therapist presence is the 'limited reparenting' approach (Edwards, 2017; Gülüm & Soygüt, 2022). It affords a nuanced approach beyond attuning to and meeting affect and emotional vulnerability by listening for client unmet needs, particularly those attached to core pain. This stance involves going some way (hence the 'limited') to meet the unmet developmental needs of the client in the present moment and therapeutic relationship. Thereby, it extends the corrective emotional experience and potentially, over time, updates old schemata (such as around emotional deprivation and social isolation), whilst providing a model for clients for new intra- and interpersonal ways of being through an experience that the client may have not received before. In being a 'limited parent', the therapist provides a holding environment and further promotes themselves as a new and healthier self 'object' for the client to internalise. It is important that a therapist is attuned also to situations in which they missed or did not meet self-object needs, and to be aware of the injuries and therapeutic relationship ruptures that may consequently ensue, in order that they can make efforts to repair. Table 5.1 provides a summary of some common examples of core pain, thoughts, needs, and suggested corresponding limited reparenting approaches for people with AN.

The Therapeutic Relationship when Working with Neurodivergent Clients

Neurodiversity simply refers to the reality that diverse minds and brains exist (Dwyer, 2022). Some common examples of neurodivergent neurotypes are autism and ADHD, and such neurotypes are over-represented in people with EDs compared with the general public (Cobbaert & Rose, 2023), with up to 40% of people with AN also being autistic (Nimbley et al., 2023). Neurodivergent people may experience different strengths or struggles from those with neurotypical neurotypes. In general, holding a neuroaffirmative stance (i.e. embracing and valuing all neurotypes as reflecting different ways of experiencing the world) as opposed to being informed by the medical model (i.e. seeing neurodevelopmental differences from neurotypical as being deficits based) leads to more successful therapeutic relationships with neurodivergent people (Hume, 2022). Therapists should recognise neurodivergent clients as members of a minority culture and acknowledge ingrained power dynamics (especially where the therapist is not neurodivergent, thus has neurotypical privilege), accepting in their role to adapt, show curiosity, and cultural humility (Hume, 2022).

Table 5.1 Core Pain, Associated Emotional Needs and Suggested Limited Reparenting Approaches

Broad Domain of Needs (e.g. Common Schema in Anorexia)	Core Pain	Associated Thoughts	Associated Emotional Needs	Limited Reparenting Examples
Attachment (e.g. social isolation, abandonment)	Loneliness/ sadness-based	"I am alone; I have nobody to turn to; Nobody wants to hear or can help me manage my emotions."	Love, connection, closeness	Empathic attunement, soothing, connection, reassurance, e.g. • Offering extra contact at times of distress • The use of a transitional object • Speaking to the Little Self in a gentle, caring, and holding tone (e.g. as a 'mirroring mother')
Identity (e.g. defectiveness/ shame)	Shame-based	"There must be something wrong with me. I am unlovable, broken, and defective."	Acceptance, acknowledgement, understanding	Genuinely prizing and showing the client with authenticity they are special and wanted, e.g. • Marking a special event or anniversary in some way • Expressing (genuinely felt and held) pride and/or joy at client achievements or life events • Being explicit in understanding and making practical adjustment for neurodivergent differences
Safety (e.g. subjugation)	Fear-based	"It is not safe to be myself and express my needs."	Relational safety and protection, freedom to express valid emotions	Guiding and encouraging expression of the Self and offering appropriate protection, e.g. • Advocating for a client's needs with other team members or family • Hearing and encouraging emotional expression with curiosity and interest • Encouraging unseen or under-expressed parts of the self, such as playfulness and child-like fun, spontaneity, enjoying things together

Being neurodivergent can influence relational styles and communication preferences and it has been suggested that the development of a therapeutic alliance between a therapist and clients where they are of different neurotypes might require adaptations to a therapist's standard practice (Jellett & Flower, 2024). This can include language (e.g. autistic people tend to take things in their literal sense and have reduced conceptual reasoning) or non-verbal communication (e.g. preferring to avoid eye contact). Neurodivergent clients can struggle with questions with too many clauses or concepts, so these should be avoided. There may be levels of inattention or a need for movement during the course of a standard 50-minute therapy session. Difficulties with reading or writing and/or strong preference for a particular learning style such as visual learning or having a slower processing speed may be present. Autistic people report a preference for practical considerations such as therapy in low-stimulus environments, at consistent days/times and location (Lipinski et al., 2019). Explicitly exploring and embracing what these factors bring to the therapy environment for each unique client creates a sense of safety for autistic adults (Hume, 2022). Furthermore, it enables a practical accommodation of sensory and cognitive needs to ensure clients can fully access and engage with the work. In short, there is a need for balance of "tolerable nurture and tolerable structure" (Bowers & Widdowson, 2023, p. 39).

Of note is that neurodivergent and neurotypical adults can differ in overall emotional expressivity (Foster et al., 2024) and autistic people report that neurotypical people may not accurately read their emotions (Camm-Crosbie et al., 2019). Thus therapists should adjust expectations of what emotions may look like or how they might be expressed. Further complicating this is that neurodivergent people commonly mask their authentic selves as a social strategy – to fit in or to avoid stigma. Masking can result in disconnection from a true sense of identity with a negative impact upon well-being (Miller et al., 2021). Masking can be seen as akin to using coping modes in social interaction (see 'Formulation and Conceptualisation', this chapter, for further discussion of coping modes). Unmet developmental needs for authenticity, sense of safety, recognition, and self-consistency (in understanding who they are) are greater for neurodivergent people due to experiences of living in a world developed for a neurotypical neurotype and associated judgement for being different (Bolton, 2023; Bowers & Widdowson, 2023). Thus, neurodivergent people with EDs are perhaps at even greater risk of difficulties associated with a 'lost emotional self' and related core pain, as outlined in the SPEAKS theory and conceptualisation. Therapeutic relationship values such as unconditional positive regard, acceptance, and attunement powerfully counter the messages neurodivergent people have internalised (Bolton, 2023) and the therapeutic relationship can be the first time the client has felt safe enough to be their 'Real Self' (Bowers & Widdowson, 2023). The most important variables seen as pivotal to therapeutic relationship-building by neurodivergent clients are authenticity, empathy, and feeling liked (Hume, 2022) with a therapist who is stable, dependable, and protective (Bowers & Widdowson, 2023).

In summary, taking a neuroaffirmative, open, and curious stance and establishing a client's unique needs and preferences in the therapeutic relationship is crucial when working with neurodiveregent clients. A fundamentally different approach does not appear to be needed for relationship-building – doing more of the same is indicated, such as taking a position of enhanced practice of empathic attunement, presence and 'limited reparenting'.

Establishing Goals

Goals are important in SPEAKS. It has been found that failure to establish agreed goals early (by session 5) in short-term experiential therapy like SPEAKS is associated with poorer outcomes (Watson & Greenberg, 1996). Shared agreement on *what* to work on and *how* that work is achieved involves explicit and collaborative discussion between therapist and client. Brief psychoeducation about both EDs and the rationale for taking an emotion focus in therapy, alongside some description of the tools of therapy (e.g. imagery, chair tasks) are recommended. Following this, some early behavioural change and agreed ED management and monitoring should be explored (within the scope of what currently feels possible for the client whilst also balancing this with risk). In this section we briefly cover what *psychoeducation* and *risk and eating disorder management* include, as well as some suggestions for approaching *goals*.

Psychoeducation

Clients often have a general awareness that they struggle in the realm of emotions and therefore the approach of SPEAKS is usually met with a degree of interest and curiosity. It can be helpful to share an evolutionary perspective on emotions, such as that they help us survive and thrive, and the issues that arise when we struggle or block our emotional world. This can happen when emotions: (1) get out of balance (we feel them too much or too little), (2) we cover up one emotion with another (sometimes the most important emotion is hidden under layers of other emotions caught up in our ways of coping), (3) we miss a crucial piece of information about the emotion we are feeling, or (4) we get stuck in emotional ghosts from the past, leftover from traumatic early experiences and that don't belong in the present (Elliott & Greenberg, 2021). Elliott & Greenberg (2021) also recommend the sharing of some sayings that usefully reflect some of the theory and processes underpinning EFT, and thus SPEAKS, such as: "You can't leave an (emotional) place until you arrive" and "Every feeling has a need, every need has an action." It is important that all clients have permission to ask questions and seek clarification here and throughout therapy, and neurodivergent clients may need explicit reassurance to do this (Bowers & Widdowson, 2023).

It is also valuable to provide a compassionate framework for the emergence of parts of self by discussing core emotional needs (Lockwood & Samson, 2020).

For some clients who have endured extreme neglect or abuse in childhood there may be minimal awareness even at a cognitive level of the basic needs of a child. It is important to weave in some appropriate psychoeducation so clients can gain awareness of areas where their needs were chronically unmet, but also where there may had been islands of nourishment of need and therefore a degree of protection (such as when some emotional nurturance is afforded, for example, by a particular person in the child's earlier life). This sets a normalising context for describing how core needs if chronically unmet in childhood contribute to the development of belief systems, influencing how people think, feel, and behave (schema), and coping modes – which are simply, the most adaptive ways to cope at the time and context in which they developed. Furthermore, when we progress to the stage of formulation, we can return to the issue of core emotional needs, noticing how patterns of unmet need can fuel a critic ("I must be 'bad' that I am always alone and unloved"), as well as contribute to reliance on coping modes (such as a detached part to dissociate from the critical attack). Ultimately SPEAKS aims for clients to relate to themselves and others in ways that support their emotional needs being met, and so we return to this issue of core emotional needs throughout SPEAKS.

Psychoeducation around the physical and psychological impact of EDs can also be provided here. This should include health consequences of unchecked EDs, nutritional health facts and information, and ways in which EDs are perpetuated (e.g. diets don't work, excessive restriction leads to increased binging behaviours). There are excellent texts written for clients and their families to help them better understand eating disorders and how they best support their loved one (Treasure & Alexander, 2013; Treasure et al., 2016). It should be noted that for those who are lacking in motivation or therapy engagement at this stage, psychoeducation around eating disorders may not be helpful or can leave the client feeling misunderstood (Gregertsen et al., 2017) and this information may be usefully revisited in Phase 2.

Risk and ED Management

It is important to stress that although SPEAKS proposes a focus on a core emotional change process for recovery from an eating disorder, this does not mean that eating, weight, shape, and risk management are ignored. From early on in therapy attention should be given to maximising early behavioural change. It can include strategies such as self-monitoring (keeping food and/or exercise diaries) and establishing a regular eating pattern, as much as is possible and realistic for now, in discussion with the client (ideally three meals a day with snacks between each meal). Sensory differences for autistic people may mean that there are foods that they have always avoided, and considering food preferred prior to onset of ED symptoms will increase the client's ability to include it into their meal plan (Loomes & Bryant-Waugh, 2021). Risk from physical health complications should be agreed to be managed using regular physical health checks, such as weekly weighing (in the first instance) and monitoring of blood tests (the frequency and results of which should be assessed and monitored by a qualified psychiatrist/phys-ician). There should be clarity over the frequency of physical health checks and any changes to plans should be explicitly discussed as far in advance as possible (Loomes & Bryant-Waugh, 2021). Weight gain (especially from a very low BMI) needs to be gradual to avoid 'refeeding syndrome' (dangerous and potentially life-threatening fluid and electrolyte shifts that can occur when a malnourished per-sons begins to eat). Symptoms of refeeding syndrome include light-headedness, fatigue, sudden changes in blood pressure and in heart rate. During recovery we would expect a 0.5–1 kg weight gain per week. It may be that for people with established AN, with a low but stable weight, any early change will be minimal. For neurodivergent people, focusing too much on change at an early stage while they are unable to sustain adaptive behaviours can increase experiences of shame (Bowers & Widdowson, 2023). However, where these discussions are empathi-cally delivered, the therapist is communicating an understanding that physical health is important and that they as therapist care about the client and want to help them stay safe. A full description of good practice guidelines for risk management in EDs is available from the National Institute for Health and Care Excellence in the UK (NICE, 2017) and from Treasure (2012).

Goals

It may be that, early on in therapy, moving on from the eating disorder is not a goal that the client wishes to consider; it may simply feel impossible or too over-whelming a prospect. Therapists would also not be looking for clients to connect too deeply with emotion very early in therapy. At this stage, setting 'mini-goals' with regular review and reflection can feel more containing for clients, espe-cially those who are neurodivergent. That said, in general autistic people report conceptualisations of recovery and thus overall goals to be notably similar to non-autistic or neurotypical people (Sedgewick et al., 2022). A good short-term goal is an agreement to work towards an empathically developed 'mode map-ping' formulation (see 'Formulation and Case Conceptualisation', this chapter) alongside some steps to stabilise risk to make space for that formulation work. Mode mapping affords an opportunity to gain a better understanding and con-sideration of how things currently play out in the client's life and if this feels a satisfying and fulfilling way to live. It can be usefully followed by a planned review (approximately session 6) to consider again the goals a client may wish to set. This ongoing and open discussion about goals, using careful pacing and con-tinuing consideration of client's preferred amount of structure, is especially rec-ommended for neurodivergent clients (Bowers & Widdowson, 2023). Additional work to move past 'stuckness' and further engage with therapy is considered explicitly in Phase 2 and this may be set as a second 'mini-goal' (Chapter 6). From there, a better understanding of the drives and difficulties of the client's current presentation will have been achieved and clearer further goals can be set for working together with core pain.

Formulation and Case Conceptualisation

We are arguably a product of our own self-multiplicity, where we are composed of many interacting, and sometimes conflicting, 'parts' (Pugh, 2021), with each part reflecting a specific constellation of feelings, thoughts, physiological experiences, action tendencies, and episodic memories. These different parts or 'modes' of being are our best attempts to manage life, and they may be more or less helpful, depending on the strategies we were taught by primary caregivers and learnt ourselves across life experiences. A self-critical part arises from beliefs about the Self, formed as a consequence of unmet need and sometimes echoing characters from the past, such as an abusive parent or a bullying experience at school. For example, the child with unmet attachment needs of love, connection, and closeness who felt chronically rejected will experience chronic loneliness, sadness and sense of abandonment, alongside a critic who tells them that they are undeserving of acceptance. People develop ways to appease or quieten the critical part of self and to protect themself from core painful feelings.

The experiencing states comprised of behavioural patterns, cognitive processes, and emotional responses which seek to protect from core pain are known in ST as coping modes (Edwards, 2022) and in EFT as coaches or guards (Elliott et al., 2004). In SPEAKS we refer to them as coping modes. Coping modes are adaptive at the time of development (in childhood), often essential to survival, yet they may be over-relied upon and too stringent in their methods for optimum well-being in adulthood. Ultimately, when our parts of self are unintegrated and not in balance this interrupts the accessing and processing of useful emotional material impacting resilience, self-efficacy, and self-agency.

There is a psychoeducational component to the case conceptualisation process. It is important that therapists make clear to clients that we are all made up of parts, all having a critic for example (on a continuum of fierceness) which has expectations for us, but which can become overly rigid or harsh or dominant depending on our exposure to critical messages as we were growing up. We all have a side that 'houses' our emotions and core pain which typically feels the pain associated with unmet need. We also have parts that have learnt to cope with unmet need and resultant pain and this links to what was available to us during our earlier lives (coping modes). It is only when the parts become out of balance and some parts become too dominant or loud, and other parts are not given a space, that problems arise. It is also stressed that there are no 'bad parts', all parts of self are welcome and are of value. People tend not to sit 'in' a mode, although they may experience significantly more contact with some parts of the self than others; rather it is natural, usual, and optimal to 'flutter' between modes. Change is more about a reshuffle or de-emphasising reliance on some parts (such as stuck coping modes) and a deepening of connection between other parts (the Healthy Adult hearing the experience and needs of the Little Self). A goal of formulation is thus to understand the parts, their origin, what their function is, how they show themselves and how they interact, as well as to appreciate some of the limitations of these ways of being and coping in current life.

This approach considers the whole person, it values and privileges an understanding of how the Self is developed, and how 'parts of self' interact. In this section, we describe how to identify and explore parts of self with a client and construct a visual '*mode map*' for clients to better understand their intra- and interpersonal patterns of relating (Green & Balfour, 2020). Case conceptualisation through the use of a 'mode map' formulation is completed early in therapy, around sessions 4 to 8. However, it remains an iterative, dynamic, and evolving process throughout therapy and will be added to as therapy progresses when applicable.

Anorexia and Parts of Self

The heterogeneity of AN and co-occuring presentations is such that there may be many diverse parts of self that are relevant to a clients presentation and which a therapist would seek to to help them identify, name, and integrate into the formulation. That said, research evidence suggests there are some parts which will emerge most commonly or more strongly for this client group. The metaphor of a theatre has been used to describe the different parts of self with some seen 'frontstage' (clear and visible), whilst others are 'backstage', even 'offstage', where they are hidden, obscured by another part or far away (Edwards, 2022). For people with AN and other eating disorders, there are often clear dominating parts at the start of therapy and others that are hidden.

Modes Likely to Be Dominating at the Start of Therapy

Coping Modes

With each client you will develop an understanding of an idiosyncratic set of self parts/modes, including many coping modes. The 'name' of the mode can be idiosyncratic and emerges from the language of the client (such as 'The Wall' for Detached Protector, 'People Pleaser' for Compliant Surrenderer or 'The Bully' for the Critic). The name can be creative as long as the therapist holds the basic theoretical primary function of each mode in mind. In ST there are considered to be three primary functions:

1) **Surrendering to** a schema or set of schema, seeing these views of the self/ world as inevitable and giving in to them, such as surrendering to a sense of 'defectiveness and shame' and believing "I am unlovable and broken and undeserving"; therefore acting in ways that reflect *self-neglect* or repeat the experience of shame and failure, such as sabotaging an intimate relationship.
2) **Avoiding activation of** a schema to block the thoughts and feelings that ensue, such as avoiding the sadness and loneliness of core pain of abandonment by

avoiding intimate relationships, in a process of *self-interruption*. This may also involve engaging a:

- *Detached Protector mode* which acts as a circuit-breaker to interrupt or block access to associated core pain, or a
- *Detached Self-soother mode* which transforms manifest emotion into something different (such as via bingeing and vomiting, using drugs, alcohol, or other perseverative activities)

3 **Overcompensation and overcontrolling** to counter a schema, such as overcompensating for core schema of 'defectiveness and shame' by *self-coercion* into working extremely hard to be 'good enough' possibly via a *Perfectionist Overcontroller mode* to keep rigid control behaviourally (such as via perfectionism) or cognitively (such as via worry, rumination, obsessionality).

The function of coping modes therefore point towards specific ways of relating to or managing underlying core pain and unmet needs for each client. Coping modes noted to be especially prevalent in eating disorder populations are Helpless Surrenderer (giving and depending on others entirely for rescue or care, such as seeking hospitalisation so that the decision to eat is no longer theirs to make), Detached Self-soother (cutting off from emotion using distracting and unhelpful soothing behaviours, including ED behaviours such as excessive exercise or binging) and Compliant Surrenderer (people-pleasing and meeting other's needs, even at the persistent expense of one's own) (Simpson et al., 2018).

Eating Disorder Part

There is of course also the Eating Disorder Part (EDP) which can be framed as a coping mode or Critic; typically in SPEAKS the EDP is 'held' in both. The Critic espouses beliefs about the self, core messages like, "You are taking up too much space .... too fat ... too much ... no good" with the coping mode acting on the messages and trying to buffer the impact on the feeling part (e.g. Little Self) via an Overcontroller part that may restrict to block the feelings or a Self-Soother part that may transform the feelings, such as via purging. This will be very apparent at the start of therapy and may be the most prevalent mode(s) evident in the client's talk of eating and exercise plans as well as worries around weight and shape, all internalised as first-person statements ("I am fat", "I am lazy and need to exercise more", "I can't possibly even consider eating any more").

Inner Critic

The Inner Critic proffers historically-based characterological or trait-like criticisms, leading to assertions such as "I'm inferior; I'm worthless; I'm pathetic; I'm unlovable", which the client seeks to 'fix' or ameliorate via ED achievements and goals, alongside using coping modes. Attacks by the broader Critic therefore trigger the EDP into action. They also trigger the stuck core pain of shame of perceived inadequacy or the sadness of feeling lonely and abandonment. Therefore, accessing and working with the Inner Critic helps therapy to move beyond the symptom-level to the core pain.

Modes Less Obvious at the Start of Therapy

Little Self

The 'Vulnerable Child mode' of ST is called the 'Little Self' in SPEAKS. It is conceptualised as housing the core painful emotions (primary maladaptive emotions) based on past memories of developmental unmet need (schema), that are typically shame-based, sadness/loneliness-based or fear-based. Thus accessing the emotional experience of the Little Self is central to transforming and healing core pain. For people with AN, the Little Self is often partially dissociated and sometimes non-verbal. It can be blocked out by a coping mode taking 'centre stage' and as such is "hidden behind a wall of survival" (Edwards, 2022).

The Healthy Adult

The Healthy Adult was originally coined in ST as a mode typically considered to be distinct, which offers an overseeing or meta-role for the other 'parts of self'. Its functions include the developing capacity to "see previously unseen possibilities for action" which instils hope, creativity, flexibility, and self-agency (Salicru, 2023, p. 939). This part engages in 'positive treatment of self' including self-care, self-acceptance, self-empathy, and self-direction. In SPEAKS, the Healthy Adult is seen as a distinct mode, but core to its functioning is a psychologically adaptive relationship with the Self that emerges over the course of therapy (Cf. Oldershaw and Startup, 2020). However underdeveloped and unintegrated or 'off the stage' the Healthy Adult may be during Phase 1, it is considered absolutely key to the SPEAKS model of change and is named and worked with from the outset. Clients might recognise a Healthy Adult part of themselves as something shut off and which they would like to embrace more, but it is important the Healthy Adult is not idealised as a 'perfect' Self that becomes unrealistic and unachievable, which is a risk for this client group. The SPEAKS approach to the Healthy Adult as something that is named, but naturally emerges and is strengthened through the transformation of emotional pain, positions it from the start as having a close connection with the Little Self and being integrated within other parts, thus establishing its authenticity.

The 'Real Me'

The 'Real Me' emerged from SPEAKS development work as a state associated with recovery recognised by people with lived experience of AN. In SPEAKS, it does not reflect a part per se, or an 'idealised self', but rather the whole reconfigured and integrated richness of self, still containing coping modes and the Inner Critic, but

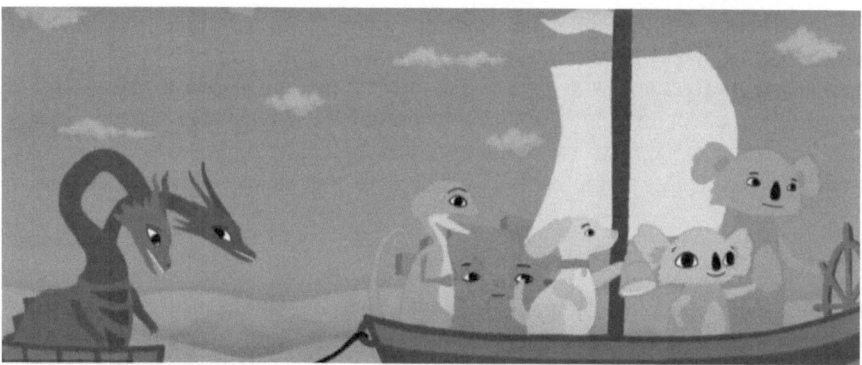

Figure 5.1 Illustration of the 'Real Me'

now led by the Healthy Adult (who can listen to and respond to feelings and needs) and the transformed Little Self (who can now safely share vulnerability and needs).

Figure 5.1 shows a still taken from the SPEAKS animation, illustrating the 'Real Me' with the Healthy Adult and Little Self at the helm (adult and child koalas), whilst coping modes (dog, wall, and lizard) and Critics including the EDP (dragons) take a backseat.

'Mode Mapping'

During SPEAKS, we first seek to help clients notice and begin to find a language for parts of self as they arise. We then utilise a 'mode' map formulation to create a concrete illustration or to 'map' with a client their 'parts of self' (Green & Balfour, 2020). It is important to notice not only the parts of self as they arise, but also how they interact. Important information for therapists is understanding how modes may block or facilitate change and interfere with relationships in clients' lives. Mode maps are transdiagnostic, they map the person not a syndrome, which can be containing for clients who present with a broader range of difficulties because often what seems like a complex array of struggles can be named and contained via interacting parts of self within this one mode map.

For some clients a 'mode map' is an intervention in itself and represents the first time they gather a meta-perspective' or overview of their self-to-self relationships. This may be especially true for clients where the Healthy Adult is less developed. It may be that they have struggled with AN for a long time, and there is an over-reliance on the AN identity making it hard to see beyond it. In this case, the mode map 'holds' the meta-awareness of the broader parts of self that eventually the Healthy Adult takes in. Mode mapping is also helpful for people who are more connected with their Healthy Adult right from the start who may require less emotion transformation of core pain and require an enhanced understanding of patterns and choices. For these people, awareness of secondary emotion and relational patterns via mapping of modes can be a significant step towards accessing primary adaptive emotion and engaging the Healthy Adult.

The visual mapping of parts affords a concrete representation of self-understanding. This approach to formulating can be particularly useful for people who are neurodivergent who can be concrete, literal, and visual thinkers and are better able to understand and use visual information (Samson et al., 2012). Clients may keep their mode maps to hand, saved on a computer home screen or a notice board for easy access and reflection on situations that emerge between sessions.

Developing the Shared Understanding

The first step to creating a 'map' of a client's parts of self is establishing a shared understanding of parts grounded in a client's narrative. During the initial sessions of therapy, the therapist will attune to the client's narrative and respond with empathy. They notice and reflect emotions as they emerge, looking out for core pain and unmet need. Importantly, the therapist is also listening out for 'parts of self' revealing themselves. The critical EDP usually reveals itself early on, as it links strongly to the symptomatic presentation. Therapists become aware of coping modes from the client's narrative and from their own observations of the client's processes. For example, after feeling the force of the Critic, a client may well 'cut off' by interrupting emotional experience altogether and become detached from emotion (conceptualised as a 'detached protector' coping mode). As such, they may talk about and 'look on' at emotions as a concept but are not truly in touch with them.

When a therapist hears a part of self, they can appropriately and gently bring it to the client's attention. In early stages, the therapist draws attention to these parts of the self in a curious and open way, speaking broadly without labelling them until a shared language has been found ("It sounds like there's a part of you that just 'cuts off' when the Critical side gives you a hard time"). The therapist is gentle with these reflections especially during the first few sessions, mindful not to overwhelm the client. Once the mode map has been drawn this provides an anchor for noticing and naming these 'parts of self' as they arise. Key to formulation is normalising the development of coping modes based on the client's history.

> It's no wonder you had to learn to detach when you felt sad, I remember you saying how your dad would shout at you until you cried, and you would hide away in your room until he calmed down. Thank goodness you could get space in your room like that, Clara. I can see why you had to cut off from pain with there being no one to comfort and soothe you. I wish you had had someone there with you to be alongside you when you felt so crushed and alone. It's like back then, you had no choice but to 'cut off' from difficult feelings. And in the present day, any hint of painful emotion sends you back to that detached place. I would love to help the 'Feeling You' to feel safe enough to be with and express how she feels. I'd love to get to know her a little more.

It is also valuable to not rely on the technical mode names, these merely signify function. Rather use client's language to fall upon a mode name. Such as for the

Detached protector – "The Wall", the Compliant Surrenderer – "People Pleaser", Vulnerable Child 'experiencer' – "Little Clara". For neurodivergent people, finding ways to name or conceptualise parts that fit with their interests can especially help ground them for the client and add understanding. For example, a client who has a 'special interest' for animals may like to name their parts after animals whose characteristics they see those parts aligning with the most. A Healthy Adult might be a compassionate lioness protective of her young, an Inner Critic – an aggressive snake, easily and quickly slithering and constricting.

Avoid using derogative names especially for child parts. Clients who endured relational trauma, for example, may call their feeling sides harsh names (such as 'Bad Me' or even 'Evil Me'). We don't want to collude with needs, feelings, or indeed any sides of the self being judged or rejected, and so we would seek to guide the client to find a gentler name, and sometimes we may need to fall upon something very simple (even functional) at this stage such as 'Feelings Side'. Later when a clearer connection between core pain and unmet developmental needs is made, this may become better understood and updated, e.g. to Little Clara.

It is important to draw attention to 'mode relationships' and to continually build awareness of how different parts of the self relate to each other and influence each other. Modes often follow each other in recognisable patterns or sequences (Edwards, 2022). These relationships are elaborated over time giving important information as to stuck behaviour and relational patterns. This all contributes to normalising self-to-self relating and building awareness of internal processes along the way, as well as highlighting stuck loops (patterns of movement between critic, coping modes, and Little Self) that may underpin behaviours that clients have named as goals for therapy. An aspect of this is considering how the ED may have interacted with parts such as creating an increased over-reliance upon a coping mode; for example, providing more ways in which a Perfectionist Overcontroller can control life (e.g. by focus on weight, calories) or a Detached Self-soother coping mode can unhelpfully soothe (e.g. using excessive exercise or binging). Likewise, consideration of how neurodivergence may have led to reliance on coping modes, such as overcompensatory coping in response to ADHD executive functioning difficulties.

Formulation is a rich and dynamic process that is built upon over time and not to be rushed through like a psychoeducational or cognitive exercise. There are many times during the process of formulating and naming modes where we pause and deepen both the experiencing of the client and our understanding of the nuances of their parts of self. From here we can make links to past experiences or updates to mode names and descriptions by adding language to the mode map or adjusting the positioning of parts in the visual map created.

Deepening an Understanding of the Parts

Deepening an understanding of parts will be achieved from exploring in conversation and narrative and during the mapping process. As required, an experiential method to deepen understanding is to 'interview' modes, to get to know their pros and cons and ultimate functions for the person (Heath & Startup, 2020). In ST and EFT this is brought to life and made more 'experiential' via the symbolism of chairs. Using chairs while a client is connected with and embodying a particular part of the self, the therapist can interview the client as the part (in this case a coping mode), first exploring patterns of its emergence (*"When did you first arrive in Clara's life? What did you do for Clara back then?"*, *"What do you do for Clara now? When are you most present?"*) and then accessing the ways in which the coping mode 'works' for the client (*"What do you help Clara manage? What do you fear for Clara if you weren't around to help her? What would life be like for her if you weren't around?"*). The client can then switch chairs and be invited to elaborate the downsides of the mode. This often takes more teasing out and careful reflection; some of the unintended consequences are not always apparent (*"What do you take away from Clara's life?"* or *"Do you ever cause Clara any problems? What are the downsides of you being so much in the driving seat?"*). When the pacing is thoughtful (to support emotional connection) and the questioning relational and with curiosity, the client can be put in touch with new cognitive insights, the pain of losses and the core pain that over-reliance on a coping mode may be masking. As such this task should be cautiously completed early on in therapy and returned to later on once emotion has begun to be expressed more openly and deeply. Indeed two chair tasks afford an opportunity for exploring this content, and extending it, by further deepening emotion to include embodying the part that experiences the losses and problems associated with the mode (See Phases 2 and 3). It can be useful to write down and share with a client these early reflections on the functions of modes, so that they can be revisited during the remapping process in Phase 5.

Creating the Map

Mapping out a client's parts of self helps to establish the 'big picture'. It involves visualising the parts and assembling them in a 'map'. This enhances meta-awareness, and highlights that less socially desirable parts or those disliked by a client do not represent the 'whole' of them, as well as outlining potential paths towards desired change (Green & Balfour, 2020). It should be seen as piecing together a jigsaw, and creating the map is likely to take a whole session, in the first instance at least, with other pieces added over time.

Visualising the Parts

The first step is to visualise the parts. This can be done as a drawing, using toys, other objects, or other creative methods as suit the client. Using toys, objects, or visual methods affords a visual and concrete understanding that is in its nature dynamic, giving the client a sense of ownership over the map and aids 'edge of awareness' and unconscious processing (Fleet et al., 2023). Furthermore, for neurodivergent clients who may be more naturally visual and concrete thinkers,

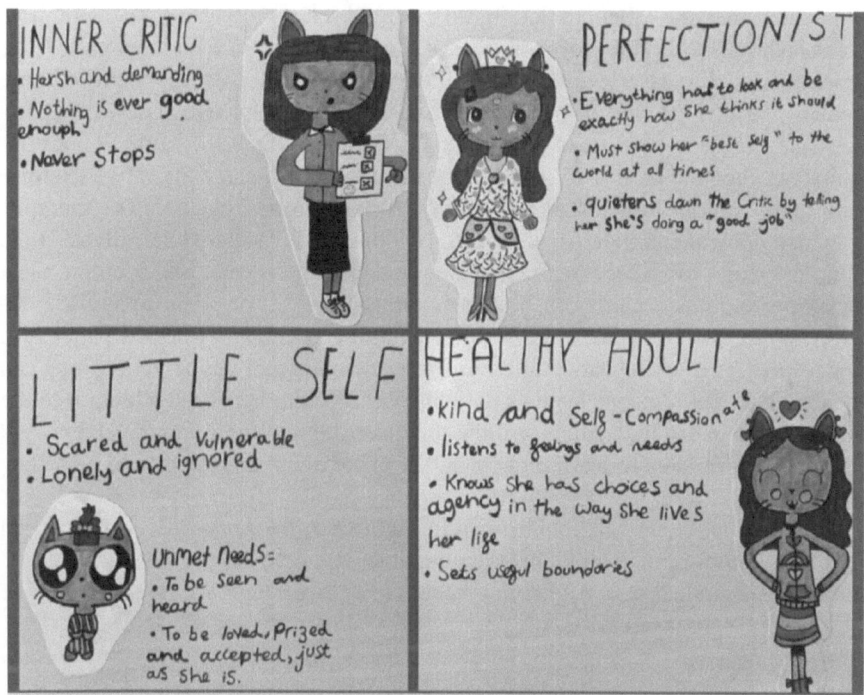

Figure 5.2 Clara's creative depiction of parts of self and associated characteristics

whilst also potentially being less inclined to symbolise and describe in words, this approach may enable a better understanding and ability to integrate what has been discussed. Visualising the parts can be discussed in the session, and/or a homework task could be for a client to create or find pictures or objects that represent the parts and bring to the next session. Figure 5.2 gives an example of one way in which parts can be creatively visualised as by Clara. The map does not need to be highly creative, however, and can be basic line drawings of shapes representing parts. If the map is being created on an online video platform with a 'whiteboard' function, a client may simply wish to choose shapes or colours to categorise parts.

Assembling the Parts in a 'Map'

If a client is using toys or objects to represent the parts, the therapist can provide these, and it can help to have a collection of toys, figures, and objects on hand for clients to choose items that represent their parts. Alternatively, a client can collect items or pictures for homework, and they should bring these to the session. Clients should be encouraged not to 'overthink' but choose items that they feel drawn to. Therapist and client can explore chosen items, affording a deeper discussion of the qualities, what drew them to that figure, what does it represent for the client, how does it show itself to the world, how does it move or interact with other parts? The client is asked to assemble the parts in the way in which they see them relating, which part is front and centre, which parts work closely together, which parts are small or far away. It can sometimes feel hard to know for sure the relationships between the parts, and it should be clear that this is an explorative exercise and there is room to adjust it later as you discover more together. The therapist can also draw attention to previous observations made in shared narratives. If the map is being drawn together rather than assembling objects, either online or at an in-person session, this can be led by either therapist or client to suit the client's approach (but remains collaborative) and can employ pen and paper or a video platform 'whiteboard' function. Here the parts and their relationships can be drawn as they emerge, such as noticing a critic chiming in and adding it to the map. However the map is created, the therapist should take a compassionate and curious stance, keen to learn more with the client about their parts and how they fit together.

In the initial client example, shown in Figure 5.3, the *Little Self* object chosen is a small mouse prone on its back, vulnerable, and defenseless. The *Inner Critic* is a ghost, goulish and frightening, able to walk through walls and enter the

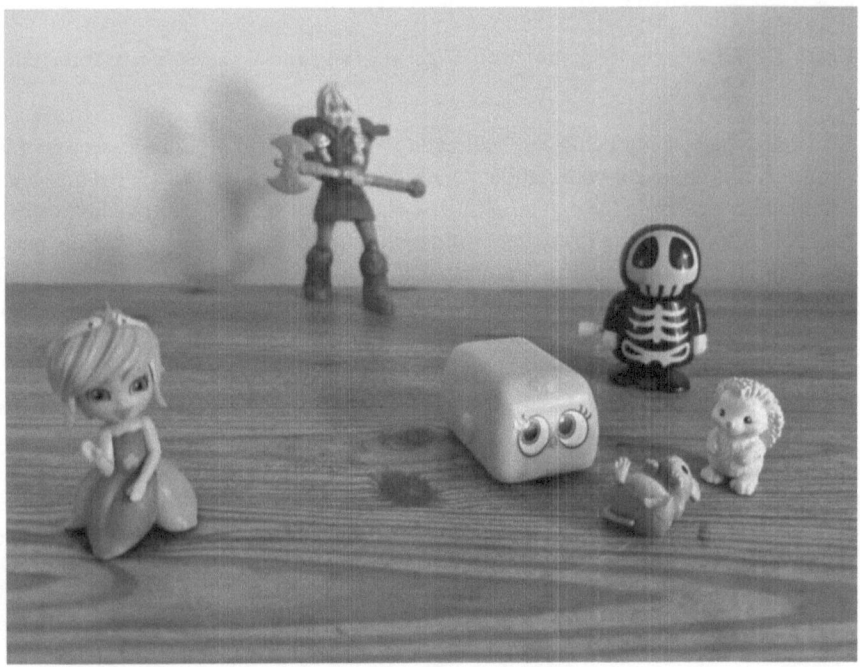

Figure 5.3 Example 'mode map' using toys/objects

client's mind at any time without warning. Standing directly over the Little Self in attempts to protect it from the Critic are an *Avoidant Protector hedgehog* (who curls into a ball and makes its world small at any time) and a *pink Detached Protector* (a box in which all emotions are crammed and sealed, looking pretty and calm on the outside). Waiting in the wings is a *Perfectionist Overcontroller* (an immaculate fairy ready to control everything with a click of her fingers). In the distance is a *Healthy Adult warrior*, who can fight for the self, but is far away and out of reach. Additional parts would be added to this map as they emerge in the therapy process.

Once the mode map is complete, the client keeps the original and the therapist takes a picture. Client and therapist are encouraged to see the map as a dynamic work in progress, being added to as more is revealed and understood during the course of therapy. Therapeutic change is continually linked back to the map during task debriefs and session summaries.

Clara's 'Mode Map'

Clara and her therapist met online and decided to construct her map as a diagram using a shared 'whiteboard' screen (Figure 5.4) with mode names chosen by Clara. During the early stage of formulating Clara noticed for the first time the role of her 'overcontroller' mode and its links to associated ED behaviours as a means to counter difficult beliefs held about herself, as well as feelings of shame. At this early stage in therapy these insights and emotions were fleeting (quickly captured and distanced from via a coping mode). Yet there was opportunity for her therapist to gently guide awareness of the richness that was unfolding in terms of the felt sense of her Experiencing Self (shame and sadness), being associated with chronic unmet need and an understandable and (to some degree) adaptive urge to distance (via the overcontroller and also detached protector coping mode, which she called the 'Emotions Squasher'). Noticing these links decreased shame and instilled a little hope and curiosity that some of her painful and difficult challenges might be worked through alongside her therapist. Clara was also open to noticing the impact of her 'Hiding Mode' (Avoidant Protector) in keeping her life small. Her therapist made the link between her unpredictable earlier life and confusing primary relationships to help Clara have compassion for her drive to retreat into avoidance or turn to 'people-pleasing' (Compliant Surrenderer) in order to stabilise her emotional world. However, she could also see that this strategy was not serving her well in the present and that another part of her (her Healthy Adult holding the needs in mind of her Little Self) longed for deeper connection to others, especially females her own age. Clara called this part Balanced Clara. At this stage Clara was able to sit with this insight, yet the pull to avoid would win through mainly because the price of feeling more and the potential of being seen as 'defective' felt too much. Its ok at this stage to just notice these mixed intentions and needs of different parts of the self and to have in mind some potential goals for therapy.

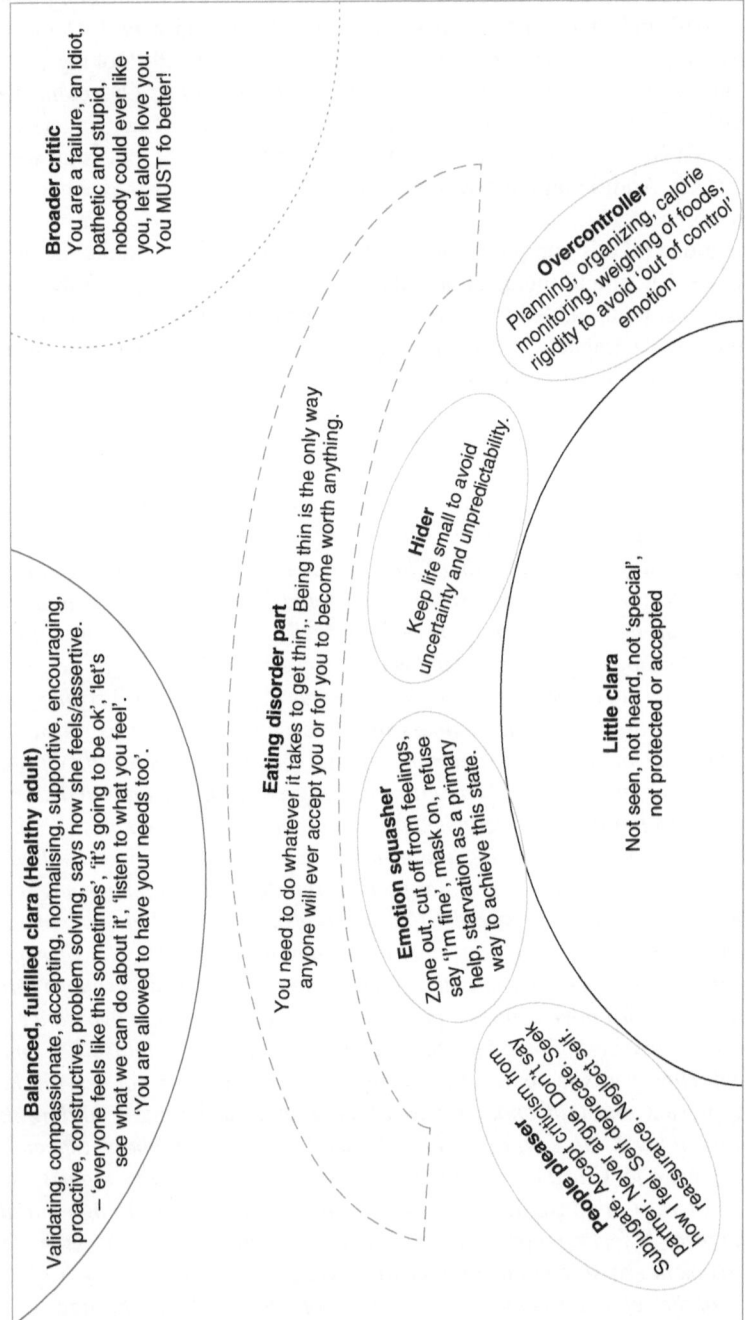

Figure 5.4 Clara's 'Mode Map'

The EDP was at the fore of Clara's reflections in Phase 1. She saw this part as dominant and powerful, feeding into her coping modes. However, she was also able to reflect on her many strengths (held in her Healthy Adult) and how on better days she knew that she could achieve a great deal if her drive and passion was channelled into something other than AN behaviours. It was emotive for Clara piecing all this together. AN can lead to clients becoming incredibly 'blinkered' and dissociated from their broader self. Thus, it is a presentation for which mode mapping can be emotional, for the first time shining a light on the many forgotten parts of the self.

References

Baier, A. L., Kline, A. C., & Feeny, N. C. (2020). Therapeutic alliance as a mediator of change: A systematic review and evaluation of research. *Clinical Psychology Review, 82*, 101921.

Banai, E., Mikulincer, M., & Shaver, P. R. (2005). "Selfobject" Needs in Kohut's Self Psychology: Links with Attachment, Self-Cohesion, Affect Regulation, and Adjustment. *Psychoanalytic Psychology, 22*(2), 224.

Bolton, M. J. (2023). De-centering neuronormativity is an imperative in humanistic psychotherapy: Towards a neurodiversity-informed, person-centered approach. *PsyArXiv.* https://doi.org/10.31234/osf.io/q2t8h.

Bourdin, D. (2023). On the analytic transference. *The International Journal of Psychoanalysis, 104*(4), 691–700.

Bowers, C., & Widdowson, M. (2023). Transactional analysis psychotherapy with clients who are neurodivergent: Experiences and practice recommendations. *International Journal of Transactional Analysis Research and Practice, 14*(1), 32–54.

Bowlby, J. (1979). The Bowlby-Ainsworth attachment theory. *Behavioral and Brain Sciences, 2*(4), 637–638.

Camm-Crosbie, L., Bradley, L., Shaw, R., Baron-Cohen, S., & Cassidy, S. (2019). "People like me don't get support": Autistic adults' experiences of support and treatment for mental health difficulties, self-injury and suicidality. *Autism, 23*(6), 1431–1441.

Cobbaert, L., & Rose, A. (2023). *Eating disorders and neurodivergence: A stepped care approach.* Eating Disorders Neurodiversity Australia; National Eating Disorders Collaboration. https://nedc.com.au/eating-disorders/types/neurodivergence/

Dwyer, P. (2022). The neurodiversity approach(es): What are they and what do they mean for researchers?. *Human development, 66*(2), 73–92.

Edwards, D. J. (2017). An interpretative phenomenological analysis of schema modes in a single case of anorexia nervosa: Part 2. Coping modes, healthy adult mode, superordinate themes, and implications for research and practice. *Indo-Pacific Journal of Phenomenology, 17*(1).

Edwards, D. J. A. (2022). Using schema modes for case conceptualization in schema therapy: An Applied clinical approach [Review]. *Frontiers in Psychology, 12.* https://doi.org/10.3389/fpsyg.2021.763670.

Elliott, R., & Greenberg, L. (2021). *Emotion-focused counselling in action.* Sage.

Elliott, R., Watson, J. C., Goldman, R. N., & Greenberg, L. S. (2004). *Learning emotion-focused therapy: The process-experiential approach to change.* American Psychological Association.

Fleet, D., Reeves, A., Burton, A., & DasGupta, M. P. (2023). Transformation hidden in the sand; a pluralistic theoretical framework using sand-tray with adult clients. *Journal of Creativity in Mental Health*, *18*(1), 73–91.

Foster, S. J., Jones, D. R., Pinkham, A. E., & Sasson, N. J. (2024). Facial affect differences in autistic and non-autistic adults across contexts and their relationship to first-impression formation. *Autism in Adulthood*. https://doi.org/10.1089/aut.2023.0199.

Geller, S. M., & Greenberg, L. S. (2023). *Therapeutic presence: A mindful approach to effective therapeutic relationships*. American Psychological Association.

Green, T. C., & Balfour, A. (2020). Assessment and formulation in schema therapy. In G. Heath & H. Startup (Eds.). *Creative methods in schema therapy* (pp. 19–47). Routledge.

Greenberg, L. S. (2017). Emotion-focused therapy of depression. *Person-Centered & Experiential Psychotherapies*, *16*(2), 106–117. https://doi.org/10.1080/14779 757.2017.1330702.

Greenberg, L. S. (2021). *Changing emotion with emotion: A practitioner's guide*. American Psychological Association. https://doi.org/10.1037/0000248-000.

Gregertsen, E. C., Mandy, W., & Serpell, L. (2017). The egosyntonic nature of anorexia: An impediment to recovery in anorexia nervosa treatment. *Frontiers in Psychology*, *8*, 2273.

Gülüm, İ. V., & Soygüt, G. (2022). Limited reparenting as a corrective emotional experience in schema therapy: A preliminary task analysis. *Psychotherapy Research*, *32*(2), 263–276.

Heath, G., & Startup, H. (2020). Creative methods with coping modes and chair work. In G. Heath & H. Startup (Eds.). *Creative methods in schema therapy* (pp. 178–194). Routledge.

Hume, R. (2022). Show me the real you: enhanced expression of Rogerian conditions in therapeutic relationship building with autistic adults. *Autism in Adulthood*, *4*(2), 151–163.

Jellett, R., & Flower, R. L. (2024). How can psychologists meet the needs of autistic adults? *Autism*, *28*(2), 520–522.

Kohut, H. (1977). *The restoration of the self*. University of Chicago Press.

Lipinski, S., Blanke, E. S., Suenkel, U., & Dziobek, I. (2019). Outpatient psychotherapy for adults with high-functioning autism spectrum condition: utilization, treatment satisfaction, and preferred modifications. *Journal of Autism and Developmental Disorders*, *49*, 1154–1168.

Lockwood, G., & Samson, R. (2020). Understanding and meeting core emotional needs. In G. Heath & H. Startup (Eds.). *Creative methods in schema therapy* (pp. 76–90). Routledge.

Loomes, R., & Bryant-Waugh, R. (2021). Widening the reach of family-based interventions for anorexia nervosa: Autism-adaptations for children and adolescents. *Journal of Eating Disorders*, *9*, 1–11.

Miller, D., Rees, J., & Pearson, A. (2021). "Masking is life": Experiences of masking in autistic and nonautistic adults. *Autism in Adulthood*, *3*(4), 330–338.

NICE. (2017). *Eating disorders: Recognition and treatment*. NICE Guideline (NG69). National Institute for Health and Care Excellence. https://www.nice.org.uk/guidance/ng69/resources/eating-disorders-recognition-and-treatment-pdf-1837582159813.

Nimbley, E., Gillespie-Smith, K., Duffy, F., Maloney, E., Ballantyne, C., & Sharpe, H. (2023). "It's not about wanting to be thin or look small, it's about the way it feels": an IPA analysis of social and sensory differences in autistic and non-autistic individuals with anorexia and their parents. *Journal of Eating Disorders*, *11*(1), 89.

Oldershaw, A., & Startup, H. (2020). Building the healthy adult in eating disorders: A schema mode and emotion-focused therapy approach for anorexia nervosa. In G. Heath & H. Startup (Eds.). *Creative methods in schema therapy* (pp. 287–300). Routledge.

Pugh, M. (2021). Single-session chairwork: overview and case illustration of brief dialogical psychotherapy. *British Journal of Guidance & Counselling*, 1–19.

Roediger, E., & Archonti, C. (2019). Transference and therapist–client schema chemistry in the treatment of eating disorders. In S. Simpson & E. Smith (Eds.), *Schema therapy for eating disorders* (pp. 207–220). Routledge.

Rogers, C. R. (1975). Empathic: An unappreciated way of being. *The Counseling Psychologist*, *5*(2), 2–10.

Salicru, S. (2023). The healthy adult in schema therapy: Using the octopus metaphor. *Psychology*, *14*(6), 932–951.

Samson, F., Mottron, L., Soulières, I., & Zeffiro, T. A. (2012). Enhanced visual functioning in autism: An ALE meta-analysis. *Human Brain Mapping*, *33*(7), 1553–1581.

Sedgewick, F., Leppanen, J., Austin, A., & Tchanturia, K. (2022). Different pathways, same goals: A large-scale qualitative study of autistic and non-autistic patient-generated definitions of recovery from an eating disorder. *European Eating Disorders Review*, *30*(5), 580–591.

Simpson, S. G., Pietrabissa, G., Rossi, A., Seychell, T., Manzoni, G. M., Munro, C., Nesci, J. B., & Castelnuovo, G. (2018). Factorial structure and preliminary validation of the Schema Mode Inventory for Eating Disorders (SMI-ED). *Frontiers in Psychology*, *9*, 314057.

Treasure, J. (2012). *A guide to the medical risk assessment for eating disorders*. South London & Maudsley NHS Foundation Trust. https://www.kcl.ac.uk/academic-psychia try/assets/guide-for-medical-risk-assessment-december-2012.pdf.

Treasure, J., & Alexander, J. (2013). *Anorexia nervosa: A recovery guide for sufferers, families and friends*. Routledge.

Treasure, J., Smith, G., & Crane, A. (2016). *Skills-based caring for a loved one with an eating disorder: The new Maudsley method*. Routledge.

Watson, J. C., & Greenberg, L. S. (1996). Pathways to change in the psychotherapy of depression: Relating process to session change and outcome. *Psychotherapy: Theory, Research, Practice, Training*, *33*(2), 262.

Winnicott, D. W. (1960). The theory of the parent-infant relationship. *International Journal of Psychoanalysis*, *41*(6), 585–595.

Chapter 6

Phase 2

Seeing through and Moving past the Façade

Chapter 6 outlines core processes involved in Phase 2 of Specialist Psychotherapy with Emotion for Anorexia in Kent and Sussex (SPEAKS). The primary aims of this phase are to further reduce eating disorder (ED) behaviours and enhance motivation for engagement with therapy and with emotion. At this point in therapy, we begin to see clients move beyond the surface level of the symptom narrative, coping modes and secondary emotion and towards glimpses of connection with primary emotion and core needs. The therapeutic journey is now one of *changing relationships with emotion* and invites a willingness to connect with affect. Several methods are proposed for conceptualising and *working with 'stuckness'* which is inevitable during this phase. To move beyond the symptomatic narrative and open a channel to access core pain, dialogues with the Eating Disorder Part (EDP) are initiated in *working to move past symptoms to underlying processes*.

Changing Relationships with Emotion

People with anorexia nervosa (AN) commonly have developed unhelpful and negative beliefs about emotion (Kyriacou et al., 2009; Oldershaw et al., 2012), with higher levels of negative beliefs correlating with self-reported emotion avoidance (Oldershaw et al., 2012). Negative beliefs about emotion (e.g. "If I feel emotions they will become so overwhelming that I won't be able to cope"; "Emotions are pointless"; "Emotions are frightening") can therefore be linked to the development and persistent activation of a coping mode of 'Detached Protector' and the interruption of emotional experience resulting in emotions being blocked partially or entirely from the client's awareness. A valued aspect of AN itself is reported to be its capacity to distract from emotion via cognitive distractions, (worry, rumination, calorie/weight hyperfocus) and reduction in physiological experience of emotion with starvation (Brockmeyer et al., 2012; Startup et al., 2013).

This emotional avoidance is argued to underpin the maintenance of the 'lost emotional self' and anorexia (Oldershaw et al., 2019). Indeed, those recovered from AN have significantly more positive beliefs about emotion than those currently unwell (Oldershaw et al., 2012). In SPEAKS development work (see Chapter 1), we spoke with people who were recovering from anorexia, and they told us that an important

DOI: 10.4324/9781003468349-8

step towards recovery was shifting their beliefs about emotions and becoming less avoidant of them in order to engage fully with life (Drinkwater et al., 2022).

SPEAKS thus argues that building a life and identity away from an eating disorder starts with beginning to change relationship with emotions from something to be avoided to something that is seen as valued and helpful. SPEAKS aims to help people understand emotions as useful guides in their lives and as intrinsic to their identity. Later in therapy this involves connection with and resolution of core pain, but the process begins as described here by slowly growing *emotion awareness*, supported by therapists acting as 'Emotion Coaches'.

Emotion Awareness and Emotion Coaching

Helping clients to foster a new relationship with emotion is a continuous therapeutic goal occurring throughout and across therapy. It will begin in the very first session as the attuned therapist shows curiosity and openness to the client's emotional experience for the first time. For people who are so practised at ignoring, distracting, escaping from, and suppressing their feelings, this can be a new and surprising experience. Whilst what is described in this section can be applied from the outset, here in Phase 2, the therapist moves more explicitly to foster a client's emotional awareness. Enhancing emotional awareness involves focusing on the body and internal felt sensations to bring evoked emotions into awareness so they may be identified, labelled, and expressed. It is detailed, nuanced, and accepting, a process of uncovering "this is where you are right now" in the moment-to-moment client experience. By becoming more aware of evoked emotions, clients can hold, own, and use the experience – now they are having an emotion, rather than the emotion 'having them' (Greenberg et al., 2007). This subtle but important shift also aligns with the goals of internal reconfigurations in therapy, such as the Healthy Adult who can listen to the Little Self with agency and willingness, resulting in enhanced self-regulation of emotion.

Increasing awareness of emotions may be particularly complex for people with anorexia and/or those who are neurodivergent. Alexithymia meaning literally 'no words for mood' (Lesser, 1981) captures the inability to describe and/or recognise one's own emotions. Significantly higher levels of alexithymia have been observed for autistic individuals (Kinnaird et al., 2019) and for people with eating disorders (Westwood et al., 2017) than in the general population. Greater alexithymia is associated with increased eating disorder symptomatology (Saure et al., 2022). Without words for emotion and confusion at times over social situations and the meaning or recognition of social nuances, neurodivergent people are especially at risk of perceiving their emotions and needs as wrong or inappropriate, and high levels of emotion suppression are observed for this group (Samson et al., 2012). Developing emotional awareness can thus be an effortful process, for those with anorexia and/or neurodivergent people. It may need to be slow with sufficient space for the client. Yet, this groundwork is essential to the therapeutic goals of adaptive emotion processing.

Therapists as 'Emotion Coaches'

Therapists can be thought of as 'Emotion Coaches' as they support clients in their *discovery of emotion* – becoming aware, tolerating, symbolising, making sense of it and locating it in relation to parts of self (Greenberg, 2004; Warwar & Ellison, 2019). The Emotion Coach encompasses a style that is 'leading and following' (Greenberg, 2010); staying close to the client's 'live' experience and staying within the 'proximal zone of development' (Eun, 2019), whilst also gently guiding them in emotional processing to locate each next step as it comes into view. Here we broadly break down the role into two main functions – 'Attending Within' and 'Moving Through' – although the experienced Emotion Coach will be working fluidly across both. As well as its general application in session, this approach can afford deepening of emotion in task work and help clients specifically presenting with unclear feelings (Elliott et al., 2004).

Attending Within

Coaching clients to attend within is key to working emotionally in therapy. This internal reflection is an underlying process occurring throughout therapy and across tasks. Having one's emotions symbolised, named, and responded to with empathy by a therapist leads to relief and comfort and has a soothing and regulatory function in the moment. This process seems particularly relevant given the role of emotion regulation in mediating the relationship between alexithymia and eating disorder symptoms (Muir et al., 2024). It also instils a process that will continue beyond therapy and is key to developing self-soothing and self-regulation and to using helpful emotion information as a guide to life. Post-therapy it will reflect how the Healthy Adult attunes to the Little Self. At this stage in therapy, the process of internalisation of new healthy 'objects' is just beginning, and it is the therapist who is attuning to a client's Little Self. The process requires the attuned therapist stance outlined in Phase 1 and involves five key steps.

(1) **Attend inwards** (Can you turn your attention inwards?): Encourage clients to non-judgementally turn their attention inward to their internal feelings, physical sensations, meanings, intentions, needs, memories. The therapist responds by communicating empathic understanding and exploration (Elliott et al., 2004) such as *experiential and exploratory questions* (e.g. "What is it like inside?", "Where in your body is this feeling?"), empathic questioning and silence in an attitude of 'receptive waiting' to allow the person to reflect on their internal felt sense. The therapist should be aware that some clients will find focusing uncomfortable, strange, and difficult to complete, and perhaps even frightening. They may find that parts of self intrude on their ability to complete the task. The Critic can get loud ("This is stupid, you are stupid for thinking your feelings are important"), or coping modes such as Detached Protector interrupting the experience of emotion ("Don't feel this. It is too

uncomfortable; don't go there"). The therapist should help the client notice these interruptions and approach these reactions with patience, validation, understanding, and supportive containment, encouraging the client to put them aside and to stay with the feeling. Therapist communication of their empathic understanding can support clients here. *Empathic affirmation* is a communication to hold the painful or difficult emotion in the therapeutic space between you, using a validating, supporting, or sympathetic response ("That's really hard, I can see how you struggle with that"). *Empathic attunement* to reflect clear tracking a client's experience can involve mirroring their body language, using responsive facial expression or repeating back short phrases. *Empathic reflection* involves saying what you see to reflect the most central, poignant or main point of the client's experience ("I see how your shoulders slump. It's so heavy ..."). Alongside therapist responses, encouraging clients to draw on existing or develop further means of tolerating emotions such that they can stay with the experience here can be beneficial (See Chapter 7).

(2) **Search inside** *(Can we capture it?)*: Find words, images, concepts or memories that capture and symbolise this emerging inner experience. Once the client has been able to settle on their felt sense and seems ready, the therapist seeks to help them to find words, labels, metaphors and/or images that capture it (avoiding any interpretation).

- "What is the quality of the feeling?"
- "What words, phrases or images come out of this feeling?"

Therapists can check in with the client whether the word or image emphasised fits their feeling ("Does that capture it?"). And if not, what might fit better ("Can you ask the feeling, 'What are you then?'"). If the client seems very stuck, the therapist might offer a metaphor or description (e.g. "When you were talking about that loneliness and uncertainty, I had this image come to mind of somebody fumbling around alone in the dark .... does it feel something like that ....?). Ultimately, however, the client decides if this fits or not, and it will be clear from their response whether it does. Any hesitancy or uncertainty from the client (e.g. "I don't know") should be taken to mean no, and exploration continues.

(3) **Actively express** *(Tell me more about it)*: Expressing the experience can rely on verbal or non-verbal expression and may require additional guiding from the therapist to support the clients in finding the right expression that 'fits'. Now that the feeling has been symbolised and expressed, the meaning made can lead to a change, usually in the form of a physical shift, a 'lightness', contentment, or relief. The therapist enquires whether the feeling is the same now or whether there is a shift. They support the client in finding words for any new emotional experience.

(4) **Have the expression heard** *(I hear you)*: The expression of the emotional experience in the warmth and acceptance of the therapeutic relationship enables clients to learn that they (and their emotions) can be accepted and valued

just as they are, that their experiences are worthwhile and meaningful, that it is safe and valid to have feelings, and also that feelings can have important meanings if you take a moment to look. This is the beginning of a new relationship with emotion, which when repeated over time can lead to new more helpful beliefs about emotion.

(5) **Reflect** *(What can we take from this? And Where from here?)*: Connecting with emotion can bring a curiosity about where the feeling came from, especially if there was a feeling shift; why this deep sense of loneliness or anxiety? Here the Inner Critic or the EDP may become apparent as well as links between the core pain and unmet needs of the Little Self, e.g. the loneliness may be accompanied by feelings of shame and a sense that the client feels they cannot be accepted by others, that they will always be rejected because they are not enough. Carrying forward can mean using this as a marker for a new task (e.g. Two chair task with the EDP, see this chapter), thinking what this means for the client's life outside of the session, or linking to the client's mode map and adding newly revealed emotions to the part of self they are linked to (e.g. adding core painful emotions to Little Self).

Moving Through

In addition to hearing and holding a client's emotions, therapists will encourage and guide clients towards new emerging emotional experiences, perceptions, or needs. This is partially inherent in task delivery and instructions (e.g. instructing the EDP: "Tell her exactly what will happen if she tries to make changes to her eating."). However, it is also needed to guide clients within their internal processes to emotion of the edge of awareness. Here it is done with empathy, openness, and curiosity, and not with an explicit or fixed pursuit of a pre-decided goal. It is importantly further facilitated by the therapist's empathy and how it is communicated. Therapists can select from a range of empathic responses to best facilitate the client process (Elliott et al., 2004). Elliott et al., (2025) describe the process like that of sailing a boat, attuning to the wind, its strength and direction, then maintaining tack, adjusting the sails to change tack, or taking a moment to drift, as will best befit progress. Importantly, a therapist is responsive to how a client receives their empathic response and adjusts their approach accordingly (Elliott et al., 2023).

Types of empathic responses therapists will most commonly use are those which bring client's attention to something just out of awareness or heighten the felt sense of the experience. *Exploratory reflections* are tentative and wondering and open ended to encourage the client to look further ("And it just leaves you feeling so …?"). *Empathic conjectures* are tentative guesses at immediate client experiences that are perhaps on the edge of client awareness or which they have been unable to say aloud yet, and which therapist attunement alerts them too ("When you say this, you feel angry …?" or "So when this part of you criticises you and says you should have done another 15 minutes in the gym it makes you feel bad … like guilty …?", "This 'bad' feeling is like a shame feeling …?"). *Evocative responses* can be used to bring client attention to implicit aspects of client's experience ("I wonder what's happening right now for you. I saw in your face something changed for a moment; what was that feeling?"), and using vivid imagery or heightening language or metaphor to increase the felt emotional sense ("It makes you want to curl into a tight tight ball and hide your face from the world") are also valuable.

Additional Considerations, Including for Neurodivergent Clients

People with anorexia and neurodivergent people report difficulty with connecting, naming, and expressing emotions, with varying reasons, but it is clear how emotion coaching through focusing can be a valuable step in working with these difficulties. People with anorexia more heavily report a distrust of the bodily self, related to their confusion over interoceptive cues and leading to behaviours such as body checking and questioning hunger cues (Nimbley et al., 2023). Autistic people describe a heightened connection with emotions but that it is an experience of "feeling the unknown" since they are often unable to identify or communicate these bodily held sensations (Nimbley et al., 2023). Autistic people have highlighted how a curious stance by the therapist who uses careful attunement and holds an understanding of how neurodivergence affects the nervous system and body reduces a sense of being misunderstood (Bowers & Widdowson, 2023). Although some evocative language can support client's connection with emotion, any figurative language should be creative and relevant to the moment. Culturally accepted phrases that can seem obscure (e.g. "you're on cloud nine") should be avoided (Loomes & Bryant-Waugh, 2021). Special or passionate interests of neurodivergent people may be a better fit to be evocative or connect to emotional experience (e.g. where animals are a special interest "it's like it vibrates inside like a lion's roar …?" or for a special interest of construction vehicles "your stomach is churning … like a cement mixer …?).

Sensory processing differences are argued to be central in autistic experiences of the world (Marco et al., 2011) and are also associated with eating disorders (Nimbley et al., 2023). In particular, autistic people are reported to have 'noisy' brain activity with excessive and constant production of information (up to an additional 42%) even at rest (Pérez Velázquez & Galán, 2013). 'Mental restlessness' characterised by mind wandering or racing thoughts is also a feature of ADHD (Martz et al., 2023). Sifting through all of the information to find the most poignant or relevant aspects or to persist with the task at hand can thus be a slower process for neurodivergent clients. Having time and empathy whilst holding the space is important. Being open to the lack of clarity is necessary and therapists may find they lean on particular empathic responses more heavily with this client group (e.g. empathic conjecture). Here the therapist communicates that the neurodivergent client is not expected to generate answers by themselves which affords a space of containment and safety. This is deemed important since being left alone to name feelings generates further anxiety and uncertainty (Bowers & Widdowson, 2023). The heightened degree of sensory information as well as difficulties processing it, require that this process is taken gently for neurodivergent people, as they reach sensory overload much more easily than neurotypical people (Oates, 2021). Autistic people may require shorter bursts of focusing work. Furthermore, working to reduce sources of additional information, such as having the client close their eyes, trying to conduct therapy in quiet spaces, or openly discussing and allowing the use of noise reduction earplugs can all help to minimise sensory overload and facilitate a focus on the internal felt sense and inner world.

Working with 'Stuckness'

People with AN struggle with motivation to change (Denison-Day et al., 2018). This may range from some ambivalence about change to being very rigid and intractably engaged in ED thoughts and behaviours. Desire for change is often mapped according to the Stages of Change model (Prochaska & DiClemente, 1983), with people with AN typically entering therapy in a stage of 'precontemplation' (do not consider current behaviour as a problem or requiring change) or at best 'contemplation' (noticing that there might be a problem, but ambivalent and still considering pros and cons). When someone has been unwell for some time and has a strong attachment relationship with the EDP alongside heavily relied upon coping modes, they become extremely 'stuck'.

The concept of a multi-parts model of the self assumes we all have parts of the self that sometimes work in opposition and sometimes 'work together'. It's also about degree and context. Using the mode map to highlight splits in the needs of different parts provides a rich and understandable account of the complexities and intricacies of motivation, meta-awareness of the parts (tracking them and their impact in everyday life) where the client begins to see they have choices, even if they do not feel ready or able to do anything differently just yet (i.e. they begin to see through the façade). So, it is less about a 'lack of motivation' than about unearthing competing needs and functions of different parts and ultimately connecting with parts that are currently hidden or underdeveloped but will be needed to help make change. In this section, we explore ways to begin to loosen and resolve clients' 'stuckness' and immobilisation in therapy. Firstly, we consider how to support clients to move past competing modes to be with underlying feelings and needs in the task 'Focusing on Stuckness'. Then we explore the emotional impact of the costs of this way of living with a goal to further access primary emotion and offer an opportunity to begin to embody the previously neglected and tentative Healthy Adult part of self in the 'Future Selves' task.

Approaches to Working with 'Stuckness'

One approach to working with 'stuckness' is to engage with the splits between parts of self that will have been elucidated from the mode map. At a basic level, this can involve putting those parts in dialogue, such as putting the part that wants to change in one chair and the part that does not in another, and then interviewing each part as you might do when building the mode map (see Chapter 5) or having each part talk to the other to explain their point of view. Yet, whilst gaining a meta-perspective and understanding of parts (as with the mode map) is valuable, this direct approach can be problematic in that the two parts usually voice their position with similar or equal strength in an overly intellectualised way. This task in particular becomes unproductive because it can be very difficult at this stage in therapy and with this client group to move beneath coping modes and deepen the task to underlying emotions and needs; the Little Self has often not yet found a voice (or is still very quiet) and coping modes very dominant. Thus while this task can be used as a less challenging or overwhelming introduction to using chairwork in therapy or can be useful for those who have yet to really think through the costs and benefits of change, the parts ultimately cancel each other out leaving a sense of 'stuckness'. In order to bypass the coping modes, SPEAKS proposes moving through this impasse to access the felt sense of being exposed to these two opposing forces; What does it feel like to be caught in this extremely difficult and 'stuck' place?

Task: Focusing on 'Stuckness'

Using imagery and maintaining the focusing stance of the emotion coach are seen as valuable means to work with and get beneath stuck patterns which can be over intellectualised. Imagery is an especially powerful tool with inherently less intellectualised mechanisms (Simpson & Arntz, 2020; Young et al., 2003). Here we describe a specific task to access the felt sense of 'stuckness' and to explore associated emotions and current unmet needs (summarised in Table 6.1).

Detailed Guidelines for Focusing on 'Stuckness'

Stage 1. Identifying the Marker and Initiating the Task – Can We Try Something?

This task is indicated when a client expresses some ambivalence, uncertainty, or resistance to making change. Equally it can be used when a client notices some dissatisfaction with the present that can be further elaborated.

Stage 2. Hear from Both Sides of the Motivation Split – What Does Each Side Have to Say?

The therapist adopts an empathic stance, wishing to hear equally from both sides of the motivation split. The stance is one of open curiosity and a genuine desire to hear from all parts without judgement or bias. Indeed, it would be quite unexpected if someone was willing or able to give up on such a relied upon way of coping easily or by reason of cognitive argument alone. The aim at this stage is to get alongside the client's narrative in its completeness and to move closer to the mixed motives of their experience.

There are different ways to engage with the client's motivation split. One way is to hear from each side. Here, you are using the chairs to differentiate the parts and heighten the connection with each side bringing them to the fore of the client's experience so the client is able to more easily access the experience of them (Elliott & Greenberg, 2021).

Another helpful way to bring the competing sides alive is to use the letter task described in the early phase of MANTRA (Schmidt et al., 2018). Here the client writes two letters in the week between sessions: One to "Anorexia my Friend" and one to "Anorexia my Enemy". The letters give the client an opportunity to describe the experience they have of anorexia as both a positive and a negative influence in their life and the associated consequences, both in the past and in the present. The completed letters are read aloud at the start of this task (ideally by client or otherwise by therapist). The therapist may reflect on the core themes and the emotional impact and invite the client to elaborate on parts of the letters or ask questions around what it was like to write them.

Stage 3. Attending to and Symbolising the Felt Sense of Being Here – *What Is It Like in This Stuck Place?*

Once both sides of the motivation split have been embodied and understood, the client can turn their attention to what it is like underneath the coping, i.e. what impact does the split have on the feeling and needs part of the self that is struggling to be heard. The therapist is seeking to help the person describe the feelings and then symbolise in some way, using metaphors or imagery.

ATTENDING TO THE FEELING

First the therapist asks the client to turn their attention inwards:

> *I am struck by what a difficult place this must be for you. On the one hand there is a part of you that tells you that anorexia is all that you can rely on and that you would be lost and useless without it; whilst on the other hand there is a part of you that so wants to get well and is desperate to have more in your life. I wonder if you can just get yourself comfortable and perhaps close your eyes, and start to look inside and focus on what it is like to be in this in place?*

FINDING WORDS, IMAGES, AND METAPHORS

Once the client has turned attention on their inner feeling, the therapist uses their stance as Emotion Coach to encourage them to go deeper and describe the 'stuck' feeling in more detail using words or images to symbolise it and to capture it in imagery (Elliott & Greenberg, 2021), such as:

Can we capture it?

- "What is the quality of the feeling?"
- "Where in your body do you experience this?"

- "What images or pictures come to mind with this feeling?"
- "Can you describe the image in detail?"

What is at the heart of it?

- (using the symbolized image as a prompt) "So what does that feel like, being on your own in the dark?"
- "What is the most important thing about this feeling?"
- "What is the worst of it?"/"What is so bad about this feeling/being here in this place?"

Where does the feeling lead you?

- "Does the feeling make you want to physically respond?
- "Is there an urge to 'do' something, like run or hide?" (exploring for action tendencies that point to a specific or possibly different feeling)

What comes with the feeling?

- "Are you aware of any other feelings that come with this loneliness?"
- "What would it feel like if it was all ok?"
- "Can you ask that feeling (or image), why are you here? Or what do you mean?"

As long as the sense of the 'stuck place' has been sufficiently evoked, clients can often come up with very vivid or clear descriptions. Clara described being stuck in a very narrow gap between two high walls, so tall that she could not see their top. All too often, Clara's experience of others was of them trying to grab at her through the wall in a way that felt intrusive, desperate, and frustrating and compounded her sense of sadness and loneliness and of being alone and misunderstood and had led to her filling all the gaps, blocking everyone out.

Clara: *I don't know … I keep coming up against a brick wall … I'm just so stuck …. I don't know where to go from here …*
Therapist: *Keep coming up against a brick wall. There's this wall and it's like right in front of you or all around you ….?*
Clara: *It's all around me, and I can't see over it. I can't climb it; there is nothing I can get a grip on …. And I keep pushing against it but it doesn't budge.*
Therapist: *What does it feel like, in this place surrounded by this brick wall?*
Clara: *It's scary and lonely.*
Therapist: *You're completely alone there.*
Clara: *Yes. But that's also comforting. There's safety here. I can't get out, but also nothing can get in. I feel like I can breathe.*

There is often a lot to explore within client's symbolisations, and they provide useful information for the developing formulation in terms of parts of self and coping modes, and also how this plays out in interpersonal as well as intrapersonal relationships.

Stage 4. Finding and Meeting the Need – *What Do You Need in This Place?*

Once the client has symbolised the place they are in, and it has been well explored, it is useful to ask, "And what do you need here in this place?". This step helps clients move on from just understanding stuckness to consider what they truly need/ want right now. It is progressed by supporting the client to meet the need in the image and can point towards moving on in some way; even if the client remains unsure of if or how they will do this. Any issues with meeting the need in the image highlights blocks and coping modes experienced by the client that can be explored ("What is in the way of making changes? What stops it being possible?").

For Clara, the need was to relieve some of the loneliness and find a safe way to connect with others, but such that it didn't feel too overwhelming. She explored the idea of moving a brick or two at waist height. She could reach through the wall when she wanted to, but it could be on her terms. Removing bricks at waist height took away expectations of eye contact or of her speaking. Using this suggestion, Clara was able to imagine removing two bricks and reaching through the wall to hold hands with her therapist, who was a quiet calming presence on the other side of the wall. Her therapist quietly noted (but did not share at this stage) how this current feeling and unmet need reflected likely developmental unmet needs (for safe connection) and core pain (lonely abandonment fear) that would be explored later in therapy.

Stage 5. Feeling Shift – *What Does It Feel Like to Have the Need Met?*

When the need has been met in the imagery, the therapist enquires about the feelings that go along with this shift in meaning. It is likely that meeting the need will lead to a shift in feeling, either a change in the intensity of the initially felt emotion (e.g. reduction in loneliness) or a new feeling (e.g. calmness and hope) will have emerged. As needed, a therapist can prompt to explore more about the new feeling.

Clara described a new feeling of calmness and hope, alongside a slight reduction in the loneliness and anxiety as she imagined the need met and the quiet connection with her therapist. Her therapist felt similar feelings, and a greater sense of connection and attunement with Clara that further strengthened their relationship.

Stage 6. Debrief and Link Back – *Can This Need Be Met in the Real World?*

These experiences, first encountered in the therapy space, can be gently scaffolded to take form in the outside life of the client. This is considered during the debrief.

(a) **Client reflects.** Client tells therapist what they notice from the task, trying to tease out any meaning made. What do they take away? What are they feeling now? There may be no change, but yet a greater clarity. Or there may have been a shift in the tension or a deeper sense of impassability of this place. Sometimes it can awaken a sadness or despair of where the client is in life right now, but within this comes new awareness of a longing or need.

(b) **Therapist deeply validates any shifts/non-shifts, praises work done and prizes emotion shared.** Any feelings are helpful and should be welcomed, acknowledged, and validated. This is an early step in encouraging the client to use their emotions and felt sense to guide them as to where they are and what they need.

(c) **Make links back to the formulation.** Reflect on any newly identified emotions and link back to parts on the map if appropriate/significant.

(d) **Decide on any appropriate action, ideas of different experiences or actions that might be tried between sessions** (keep this collaborative and client directed and scaffolded by what is possible for them at this time).

Clients can be encouraged to think about finding ways to meet the needs of the stuck place during the week between sessions. The therapist encourages responding to their emotions with gentleness and curiosity where they emerge.

Additional Considerations, Including for Neurodivergent Clients

This task has many similarities with and builds on the Emotion Coach focusing work described in this chapter by continuing to establish a link between the felt sense and the symbolisation and expression of this. Therapists should review and apply adaptations described for that work when utilising this task. Of note is that some clients may struggle with visual representations and picturing things in their mind (e.g. aphantasia) or other processing differences/preferences. Here, drawn images or words to symbolise can be utilised instead. This could also draw on special interests, a connection with nature, colours, or personal photos, as applicable.

Task: Future Selves

Addressing how EDs impact quality of life both for the better and worse and accepting inevitable losses is suggested to be important for change (Pettersen et al., 2013). Here we suggest a task to experientially build on what has been discovered in exploring the 'mode map' by inviting imagined future versions of a self who is 'recovered' or 'not recovered' into chairs and elaborating these positions using the *Future Selves task* (Pugh & Salter, 2018).

In this task there is an opportunity to talk with and move between different future envisionings of the self, as well as between them and the position of the current self. A motivation to change has been shown to be associated with identifying more

Table 6.1 Stages of Focusing on Stuckness Task

Stage	Description	Useful Therapist Prompts
1. Identify the Marker & Initiate the Task *Can We Try Something?*	Client is feeling ambivalence, uncertainty, or resistance to change and/or to therapy.	
2. Hear Both Sides of the Motivation Split – the Part That Wants to Change and the Part That Does Not *What Does Each Side Have to Say?*	• Read letters to anorexia my friend and enemy or use two additional chairs to hear from the part that wants to change and the part that does not. • Try to help client be as specific as possible about each side of the split and reasons to be for/against change.	

3. Attending to and Symbolising the Felt Sense Of Being Here *What Is It Like in This Stuck Place?*	• Attend to the feeling.
	• Find words, images or metaphors
	  - Can we capture it?
	  - What is at the heart of it?
	  - Where does the feeling lead you?
	  - What comes with the feeling?
		What are you feeling right now as we talk about this?
		What do you feel in your body?
		What images or pictures come to mind?
		What is the most important/worst part of it?

4. Finding and meeting the need *What Do You Need In This Place?*	• Client expresses the need. • Client considers how this need could be met in the imagery. • Client imagines the need being met.	What do you need here in this place? What would that look like? Can you picture this happening?
5. Feeling Shift *What Does It Feel Like to Have the Need Met?*	• Explore any shift in the experience of being in the stuck place once the need has been expressed and ideally has been met in some way.	What happens in your body now as you express this need/imagine it being met?
6. Debrief and Link Back *Can This Need Be Met in the Real World?*	Client reflects on the experience and how they feel now. Consideration is given as to how this need looks out in the real world and how it might be met there. Links are made back to the mode map as applicable.	

costs of AN and recognising its role in avoidance, compared with those not considering change (Gregertsen et al., 2017) and this is explored here. Task analysis suggests that embodying different future-selves supports decentring from the EDP and enables links to be drawn between current coping modes and ED thoughts and behaviours (Rowley, 2023). By deepening emotions to core painful feelings underlying symptomatic eating disorder behaviours and accessing primary adaptive emotion in the 'recovered self', the conflict between a future with AN and current need is more experientially and effectively explored. This is associated with more motivational change (Rowley, 2023; McKenzie, et al., 2024). Without connection to emotional experience of 'future selves', clients remain 'centred' within a coping mode and unable to connect to the Healthy Adult, such that the motivational change process breaks down. This task thus affords a structured opportunity to move between coping modes and identify the needs and values and emotion associated with each part, clearly linking coping modes to symptomatic thoughts and behaviour. Embodying the Recovered Self affords a (potentially first) opportunity to embody or imagine the previously neglected or tentative Healthy Adult self, beginning the spark of building the Healthy Adult. Table 6.2 outlines the key steps in the 'Future Selves' task, including useful therapist actions and prompts.

Motivation throughout Therapy

It is important to note that motivation is not just an issue at the beginning of therapy that can be 'fixed' and moved on from. It will wax and wane throughout. Indeed, motivation may fall to its lowest and therapy become most stuck as a client begins to deeply connect with core pain in Phases 3 and 4. A further motivational dip may occur when a client begins to see and feel a need for things to be different but still stops and interrupts themselves from taking the first steps to behavioural change and feels a deep frustration and desperation (see working to move past symptoms in the next section). The imagery identified can be revisited and reflected upon throughout therapy to describe steps or progress or difficulties, e.g. "And when that happened, it felt like those walls just got higher and higher and began to stretch even further out of sight, so you would never get over them."

The mode map is instrumental in reflecting on what is highjacking possibilities for change; typically coping modes acting as blocks or interruptions to internal process, which can then be directly worked with. For example, chair work with the Critic that says, "You always let people down and will never achieve anything so may as well give up and not even try." Or working with the 'people-pleasing' coping mode that says, "You must put other people's need first, and if you give time or energy to yourself and your recovery, other people won't like you."

Moving past Symptoms to Underlying Processes

Moving past symptoms to underlying processes involves addressing symptoms and behaviours associated with the ED and other symptom-based presentations (e.g. anxiety). When clients come into therapy, the ED thoughts and behaviours are often

Table 6.2 Stages of the Future Selves Task (adapted from Pugh & Salter [2018] and Rowley [2023])

Stage	Chair	Description	Useful therapist prompts
1. Pre-task: Letter Writing Homework	Pre-session	Clients write letters in the first person from both the perspective of themselves ten years in the future not recovered from the ED and from the perspective of the self recovered from the ED. Letters include impact on quality of life across various areas, e.g. relationships, work, health.	
2. Initiate & Introduce the Task *Tell Me, and Then Can We Try Something?*	Self chair	• Client reads letters aloud to the therapist (optimal) or requests the therapist read them out. • The process of writing as well as the content of the letters are discussed.	
3. Hearing from the Non-recovered Future Self *What Is Life Like for a Non-recovered Self?*	Non-recovered Future Self chair	• Client moves into a new chair to speak from the perspective of their *Non-recovered Self* to the *Current Self*. • *Non-recovered Self* describes specific aspects of their life e.g., relationships, hobbies, and how life feels for them. • Notice and validate secondary emotions and guilt/shame. • Encourage specific advice from *Non-recovered Self* to *Current Self*. • Notice and gently reflect advice that may come from a Critic or coping mode.	• What is life like for you? • How does life feel now? • What do you want her to know about this future?
4. Reactions and Reflections as the Current Self *How Does It Feel to Hear This Possible Future?*	Self chair	• Current Self reflects on what they heard and how it has made them feel, either talking to therapist or the Future Self. • Specificity and differentiation of feelings and emotional deepening *(may require additional chair swops)*.	• What is it like to hear this? • What happens inside? • How do you feel about this future you?

Table 6.2 (Continued)

Stage	Chair	Description	Useful therapist prompts
5. Hearing from the Recovered Future Self *What Is Life Like for a Recovered Self?*	Recovered Future Self chair	The process in Stage 3 is repeated, but as an embodied future *Recovered Self*, in a different third chair. • Listen out for self values, hopes, emotions and goals. • Listen for self-compassion or agency and encourage deepening/embodiment of these.	• What is life like for you? • How does life feel now? • What do you want her to know about this future? • How do you feel about this past you?
6. Reactions and Reflections as the Current Self *How Does It Feel to Hear This Possible Future?*	Self chair	• Client reflects on what it is like to hear from a future Recovered Self. • Deepen, specify, and differentiate feelings and emotional deepening *(may require additional chair swops).*	• What is it like to hear this? • What happens inside? • How do you feel about this future you?
6. Debrief	Self chair	(a) Client reflects. Explore any unexpected feelings, any shifts in how the client now views change and new learnings on what is blocking change. (b) Therapist deeply validates any shifts/non-shifts and praises work done. (c) Make links back to the formulation. (d) Decide on appropriate action (e.g. homework).	

consuming for them and, if we do not hold our own therapy meta-perspective, for therapists too. Although long-term change is argued to be achieved via connection with and resolution of core pain, working with ED symptoms is necessary from a risk point of view and also in order to engage with a client's current process. A key task for working with ED symptom level processes is chair work with the EDP.

Working with the EDP

The EDP can be framed as a coping mode or Critic and typically in SPEAKS the EDP is 'held' in both. As the client's relationship with the EDP changes over time, entanglement with coping modes or alignment with the Critic deepen. It is initially experienced as a 'friend' or 'protector' offering a way to cope and to avoid emotion (Williams et al., 2016). Later in the illness, the ways in which it leads to negative treatment of the self are understood and it is acknowledged as destructive and unhelpful, experienced as an 'enemy' (Pugh, 2020). Clients often hold both sides of this dichotomy and feel conflicted towards the EDP. In the 'Focusing on Stuckness' task discussed earlier in this chapter, we support clients to reflect on what it is like to live in this conflict and the stuckness it brings. People with AN describe recovery as involving a process of connecting to emotion (accepting fear of uncertainty) and separating from AN (Williams et al., 2016). Indeed, recovering a 'lost emotional self' increasingly furthered by the impact of the EDP is a key aspect of SPEAKS theory (Oldershaw et al., 2019).

Working with the EDP in SPEAKS has two core goals:

(1) To facilitate a changing relationship between the EDP and the Self such that (in the first instance) negotiating behaviour change alongside awareness and bypassing of coping modes is possible. With later use of the task (after additional work is complete) the relationship can be further modified and consolidated to highlight shifting power differentials.
(2) As a means to access a broader Critic, who fuels the EDP and provokes core pain. The recognition of the broader Critic enables a move into SPEAKS Phase 3: Deepening to Core Pain.

Task: Chair Work with the Eating Disorder Part

Here we describe a chair work task for working with the EDP. Of note is that it may look slightly different, depending where the client enters it from, and this will impact the goals of the task or where in the task one can likely progress to. Initially, where clients are very enmeshed with the EDP, the goals are to begin differentiation from it and hear it as separate. The client is encouraged to connect with the impact of the EDP on their lives, thus appreciating the disempowerment that it brings. Gradually, through continued use of the task, clients can engage with and express a counter voice, emotion is further accessed and some ED behaviour change can be negotiated. Continued use of the task here in SPEAKS Phase 2 can support an enhanced motivation to consider a Self and a life beyond the EDP. Revisiting this task in later stages of SPEAKS (e.g. during Phases 3 and 4), when the Healthy Adult is emerging, can support continued shifts in reduced power of the EDP and greater self-agency. Additional tasks (e.g. 'Saying Goodbye to the EDP', Phase 5) can consolidate the newly reconfigured sense of self (the 'Real Me') facilitated via therapy.

Using this task is like a gradually shifting seesaw; the top dog/underdog dichotomy with both poles existing even if only the top dog (the EDP) is fully within the client's awareness at the start. The task affords a gradual shift in the relative position of the seesaw poles with repeated use. At some point, the poles will be at an equal level and collaboration in the form of changes is possible. Ultimately, the goal is for the differentials to continue to shift until the client self is the 'top dog' (the Healthy Adult core self); up high, able to see the full 'self' picture.

Note that a version of this task can be used to work with other symptom-based processes, such as anxiety, depression, and obsessive compulsive disorder (see Timulak & Keogh, 2022). It is suggested that chair dialogues with symptom level distress and processes should not be the first imaginary dialogue that a client engages in due to difficulties in locating these thoughts and treatment of self (Timulak & Keogh, 2022). For those with eating disorders, the EDP is frequent and well recognised by over 90% of people with an ED (Noordenbos et al., 2014); therefore, this is likely to be a tangible, meaningful, and useful initial experiential task.

Detailed Guidelines for the ED Part Chair Work Task

Here we outline detailed notes on working with the EDP and what may emerge or be required from the therapist in each step (partly adapted from Dolhanty & Greenberg, 2009; Elliott & Greenberg, 2021; Elliott et al., 2004; Timulak & Keogh, 2022); summarised in Table 6.3).

Stage 1. Identifying the Marker and Initiating the Task – Can We Try Something?

The marker for the EDP is likely to be very evident, particularly early on in therapy and is likely to re-emerge at various points throughout all five phases of SPEAKS. Clients will talk often and in detail about weight/shape-related thoughts or behaviours (e.g. "I can't increase my food intake because then I might gain weight and that's the worst thing that could ever happen to me."). In the earlier stages of a client's presentation, the EDP may appear as a part of self that acts as a misguided coach within a coping mode, which interrupts the client's engagement with life ("If I just lose a little bit more weight everything will be fine.") and engagement with emotions, reflecting the view of emotion as unhelpful and/or frightening ("The eating disorder is so helpful to me. It protects me from engaging with feeling and I like that."). This reflects the egosyntonic nature of the EDP. As difficulties continue, the EDP reflects symptom level distress, shifting to a punitive voice that berates the client for not doing 'enough' leading to growing levels of guilt for not abiding by its rules and a sense of helplessness at the constantly moving 'goalposts' that may be reflected in the emotions or cognitions described (e.g. "I ate an extra snack on Tuesdays, and I felt so bad; the guilt was too overwhelming and not worth it. I just couldn't include the snack on Wednesday"). Prior to engaging in this current task, clients may already be able to shift from talking in a purely egosyntonic way ("I want to lose weight") to identifying the EDP specifically, framing it in the third person as a critical egodystonic voice, separate from the self (e.g. "A voice in my head tells me: 'You're so weak and pathetic for eating.'").

The therapist gently identifies this marker of the EDP being present explicitly with the client reflecting language established in the mode map as appropriate.

- "I hear that Eating Disorder part of you here. The part that tells you, you must lose weight, you should be thinner."
- "Can we explore that part a little bit more and how it affects you when it comes in strongly like this?"

The therapist seeks the client's agreement for working with this process and collaboratively sets it up. When entering the task and throughout, the therapist should aim to hold in mind whether the EDP is currently acting in more self-interruption or Critic process and notes where this may shift during the task also. This can impact the goals or interactions of the therapist as outlined.

Stage 2. Enacting the EDP – *What Does the EDP Say?*

The therapist sets up a new chair placed opposite the client's current 'Self' chair. The client is asked to move to the new chair (the EDP chair) and to enact the EDP.

- "Can you imagine yourself there and tell her some of what you were just saying? How you push her to engage in all that exercise and to keep her calories so low? You're so pathetic …"

The Critic is encouraged to be as specific and concrete as possible engaging viscerally in the task (e.g. "How do you make her feel disgusting and fat? What sorts of things do you say").

Stage 3. Self Responds to the EDP – *How Does It Feel to Hear the EDP?*

Once the EDP has expressed its opinions, the client returns to their original Self chair. When judging when to switch chairs, it can be useful to hold in mind the goals of each particular stage. Enacting and heightening the EDP (Stage 2) has the aim of evoking as deep an emotional response as possible when the client returns to the Self chair. The goal in the Self chair here (Stage 3) is to help the client differentiate the Self and the impact of the EDP from the messages of EDP, itself changing the emotional tone to focus on the toll of being on the receiving end of the powerful EDP.

INITIAL EMOTIONAL REACTION TO THE EDP

In the Self chair, the therapist seeks to explore and encourage expression of *emotion* in response, heightening the sense of attack or demand ("What is it like to hear that, to be on the receiving end of that all day?"). Note that the client's response may vary depending on the stage the EDP is at, whether it is still perceived as providing comfort and security or now experienced as hostile and controlling. Clients also may respond with thoughts or agreement and should be directed back to what it feels like to hear this EDP. The initial reaction is usually exhaustion, feeling so tired with trying to keep up with EDP demands. This can be recognised by clients even when the EDP is seen as a comfort, although motivation to change behaviour is likely to be low in this instance.

The client is encouraged to tell the EDP about this exhaustion (and/or other feelings), speaking in the here and now. The therapist reflects this here and now emotional sense of the feelings in their tone and body language (e.g. therapist sighs and rolls shoulders forwards and, using a weary tone, directs the client, "Why don't you tell her, this is just so exhausting; I feel worn down, worn out?").

DEEPEN AND DIFFERENTIATE FROM THE EDP (MOVING BETWEEN STAGE 2 CRITIC CHAIR AND STAGE 3 SELF CHAIR)

Given that people with AN describe experiencing the EDP as separate from them and simultaneously part of their identity (Higbed & Fox, 2010), the therapist will want to help the client move from an egosyntonic relationship with the EDP (self in harmony with and holding consistent values to the EDP) to an egodystonic one (the EDP being inconsistent with the client self-concept and goals) in work already begun in the working with stuckness tasks. Here, this can involve several chair swops to differentiate parts and tease out the separate messages from the EDP and the experiencing Self.

The therapist needs to be aware that this dialogue is not about facilitating a debate or intellectualising. Nor is it about the client saying what they think the therapist wants to hear in arguing back with the EDP. Rather understanding the messages and the goals of the EDP can help to reveal underlying vulnerability and maintaining processes. The therapist can explore explicit feared implications of not abiding by the EDP's rules either in the Self chair ("What's the worst thing that could happen if you don't follow her rules?") or in the EDP chair ("Tell her everything that will go wrong if she doesn't listen to you; tell her how bad it will be!"). This can reveal further symptom level concerns and drives (e.g. "I'll get fat") or deeper critical processes (e.g. "I'll be worthless, unlovable") reflecting core pain.

The therapist keeps constant attunement to core pain and opportunities for deepening to this, i.e. listening out for the Little Self. Even dialogue remaining at the symptom level, enables an important appraisal of very harmful symptom level behaviours. Therefore, it is likely to be necessary to complete this task several times with each client early on to move past egosyntonicity, enhance motivation for change and to specify and facilitate behaviour change.

Stage 4. Express the Unmet NEED – *What Do You Need from the EDP Now?*

Once the parts have been differentiated sufficiently and some aspects of the function (and ideally emotion) of the EDP have been uncovered, the client is asked to consider what it is that they need from the EDP when feeling the pressure, distress, and exhaustion it provokes.

Usually when this task has only been completed once, and particularly for clients who are still somewhat ambivalent towards change, clients will feel conflicted about asking for this and may qualify their request ("I need this, but I'm scared to have it") or keep their expression of needs very vague. This can reflect that the client has not sufficiently engaged with the costs of the EDP for the Self in an experiential way and Stages 2 and 3 may need repeating.

Clients often respond with "I need you to be quiet" or "I need you to give me a break." This expression of need in the first person, directed to the EDP, importantly strengthens a connection with the Self as separate from, and with needs that are different from, those of the EDP.

It can also be the case that clients move into a coping mode such as Angry Protector, rejecting the EDP. The attuned therapist will identify this as secondary emotion or an expression of rejection in a wish to please assumed therapist expectations that is not authentically held (i.e. reflecting a people-pleasing coping mode). In this instance, the therapist encourages the client to turn inward and check in with and connect to their feelings, then repeat the need.

Stage 5. The EDP Responds to the NEED – *Can the EDP Hear the Need?*

Once the client has expressed what they need to the EDP from the Self chair, they are invited to return to the EDP chair to respond. The therapist can direct the EDP to the key aspect of the need.

- "So Clara is saying, she is absolutely doing her best and is exhausted, and you just keep pushing and moving the goal posts. It's never enough for you. She needs a break, to be given some time off."
- "How do you respond to this? Can you see her exhaustion?"
- "How do you feel about her as she tells you this?"

The core of this stage is to assess whether the EDP can hear and respond to the separateness and vulnerability of the Self. Can the EDP let the client have what they are asking for without criticising and demanding and scaring them?

THE EDP MAY SHOW *NO COMPASSION* AND REJECT NEED

In reality, the EDP does not usually soften and pull back until there is a stronger sense of self (i.e. the Healthy Adult has begun to emerge). To shift the power differentials, individuals must first gain strength and resolve in the face of EDP attacks. It is therefore usually the Self who needs to step back from the EDP and not the other way around. Often the EDP will respond with more demanding dialogues than ever, doubling down in fear (e.g. "You must listen to me. I am the only thing you've got, the only one keeping you safe"). In this case, naming and highlighting the rejection explicitly, is followed by an enquiry around what blocks compassion and/or the function of rejection.

- "Tell her: I don't care how you feel. I am going to continue pushing you."
- "What drives you to reject what she tells you she feels and needs?"
- "What would happen if she didn't have you pushing her?"

Asking these questions can often reveal the protective and scared nature of the EDP, thereby strengthening a more assertive response from the self. Highlighting to the client these functions and needs of the EDP can enable them to consider the benefits of this in their lives and further separate. Reconsidering the continued value of the EDP and the power it has can begin the process of building boundaries and a foundation for the Healthy Adult, resulting in further initial shifts in ED behaviours (see Stage 6 below).

THE EDP MAY SHOW (PARTIAL) COMPASSION/FEAR

When this task is used later in therapy, once the Healthy Adult has emerged and is strengthening, the EDP usually responds to this. They may recognise the need and want to collaborate with the Self, but still fear the implications of this: "I see how exhausted you are and that you need a break, but I don't know how to stop this. I'm terrified of what will happen if we try." The therapist can highlight the desire of the EDP to want to change, even if there is an expressed inability to. Probing for the EDP's softened emotions toward the client underlines the potential for a more collaborative relationship, one in which negotiation is possible leading to further behaviour change.

Stage 6. Spark of the Healthy Adult – *Can the Power Differentials Begin to Shift?*

Here we want to encourage the emergence of a more adaptive internal voice in response to the EDP as the client moves to the Self chair, in contrast to previous coping mode responses; thereby laying the groundwork for an adaptive Healthy Adult voice.

SETTING BOUNDARIES

If the EDP has not shown compassion or has doubled down in the need for the client to follow their rules, the client is asked to respond to the unwillingness of the EDP to reduce their demands. Here we are probing for how far a shift in the relationship with the EDP can be supported at this stage. As such the therapist encourages the client to respond to the message of the EDP and assesses the client's ability to assert themselves.

- "How do you respond to her telling you, no, you must keep following her rules? Tell her what this will mean for you."

The client can be encouraged to react to the protective function of the EDP, if one has been established (e.g. "You say you are trying to help me, but you are actually killing me. I can't concentrate, I can't function. If you keep going, I am going to end up in hospital and I really don't want that!"). When this task is revisited in a later stage of therapy when core pain has been (at least partially) transformed, the Healthy Adult can respond more firmly and definitively (e.g. "I know you say you are trying to help me, but I don't need you in my life any more. I don't need your help, I've got this now.").

NEGOTIATION AND INTEGRATION

In either case of the EDP showing or not showing compassion, even a small shift in power differentials may enable a negotiation, such that the self can be specific in response to the EDP and in what (even small) change might be possible. The client and EDP may begin to land on common goals (e.g. staying out of hospital) and explore compromises to achieve this. By moving between the Self and EDP chair, the therapist can support the client to consider what small changes might be possible. In order to achieve this, it can be useful to highlight what the client has identified as a meaningful cost for them (e.g. "What will you need to stay out of hospital? Can you tell her?"). This can be translated into practical steps and agreement for small behavioural changes such as adding in a small afternoon snack. The client is therefore encouraged here to again express specific needs in a phase of negotiation.

Debrief

Once the task is finished, reflecting on progress or resolution is an important part of the process.

(a) **Client reflects.** Client tells the therapist what they notice from the task trying to tease out any meaning made. What do they take away? Ask the client to put into a first person 'I' statement (e.g. I deserve to try something new; I don't deserve to be spoken to like that, I have done nothing wrong; I feel a sense of relief; I feel stronger).

(b) **Therapist deeply validates any shifts/non-shifts, praises work done and prizes emotion shared.** It may be that the task only goes as far as differentiating the parts (Stages 2/3) or expressing needs (Stage 4). This is still valuable and can offer new insights.

(c) **Make links back to the formulation.** Clearly connect what has emerged to the mode map. Reflect on any patterns between modes that were newly observed during the chair task and add to the map if appropriate/significant. Highlight where the new experiences indicate change has occurred or might be needed as a focus of future work.

(d) **Decide on any appropriate action, ideas of different experiences or actions that might be tried between sessions.** Try to keep this collaborative and client directed.

Homework that builds on the negotiation is useful here. It is useful to consider with the client if and how they might add in the behaviour change agreed with the EDP during the chair task during the week. Awareness is also important. Now they have increased their awareness a client can look out for the EDP during the week to start to notice and, over time, decenter from it. This includes what happens when the agreed behaviour change is attempted.

Additional Considerations, Including for Neurodivergent Clients

Setting Up the Task

The therapist seeks the client's agreement for the task and collaboratively sets it up, emphasising that there are no expectations. Autistic clients may have a tendency to think concretely and literally, so attention should be paid to ensuring that the client understands the purpose of the task and has space to ask any questions before completing it for the first time. Autistic clients can be aware that they sometimes miss social cues and may be worrying especially about what the therapist is thinking or expecting. Explicitly enquiring about the client's fantasies about therapist expectations or reactions can be useful "I am wondering if you have any thoughts about what I might be thinking or worrying about what I'm expecting?" (Bowers & Widdowson, 2023). Self disclosure from therapists about thoughts or expectations can help build trust, alongside being straightforward and upfront whilst caring and validating (Bowers & Widdowson, 2023). The therapist can explain that they will be there to help the client, and there are no expectations about how it will go; it is just a useful opportunity to explore this internal process. Time should be spent on these reassurances for neurodivergent people who may feel the need to 'mask' or socially perform in therapy.

The client can be encouraged to differentiate by ensuring they use 'You' statements in the EDP chair (to reflect the demanding quality) and 'I' statements in the Self chair (to reflect the received impact). The therapist is supporting the client to move between inward attention to recognise and name feelings and then express them back to the EDP. This can be achieved using the stance of Emotion Coach (earlier in this chapter).

Broader Critic Processes

Whilst the EDP has often become quite disassociated from the Inner Critic, it is it is highly correlated with core critical processes (Noordenbos et al., 2014); thus theory and research suggest that it is the broader critical process and core pain driving symptom level distress. If the marker brought for this task is very critical in its nature and/or this EDP task has already been well utilised with a client, then steering towards the 'Broader Inner Critic' task outlined in Phase 3 is recommended (Chapter 7). For example, the client who has been able to recognise the function of the ED behaviours more specifically ("If I just lose a little bit more weight everything will be fine, and I will be more likable.") which highlights underlying core pain related beliefs and critical thoughts ("I am not enough.", "People will reject me.") can be guided to the 'Broader Inner Critic' task by highlighting this aspect of the narrative as the marker (e.g. "It sounds like this goes deeper than how you will look or your weight and relates to something about your sense of who you are. Can we try something slightly different here? I'd like you to imagine that deeper critic in this chair instead, the one that says there is just fundamentally something wrong with you, with who you are.").

Listen for Blocks to the Process

Clients may be able to access anger in the Self chair and get frustrated with the EDP. It can be beneficial for clients to have a new experience of emotion if anger is not something that they access easily. Therefore, it should be validated and listened to by the therapist, but the type of anger and mode it reflects must be considered. It may be the secondary anger of an Angry Protector mode, dysregulated and complaining in nature. Staying in this mode will keep the client stuck. The therapist can support them to move past it using prompts to explore and make specific client needs and the impact of not having these needs met. For example, moving past "I need you to shut up" to "When you don't shut up, I'm left feeling scared and overwhelmed and lost." This can deepen emotion to the sadness of what it is like to live like this and further shift into assertive anger. Clients may also fall into a Helpless coping mode, unable to stand up to the EDP, stuck in agreement with it and also a sense that they are helpless in life. Being evocative in amplifying the depths of the client's inability to respond to the EDP can also facilitate push back in the form of assertive anger (e.g. "Tell her, I can't stand up to you, you're too strong."). The therapist offers empathy to this position and the reparenting stance is strongly held to support soothing. This is importantly linked back to the mode map.

Moving from Phase 2 (Seeing through the Façade) to Phase 3 (Deepening to Core Pain)

Phase 2 is characterised by a slow and methodical 'chipping away' of the view that "I can't cope without this ED" and that "contact with and expression of emotions is unhelpful for me". It is seeing through the façade enough to uncover a willingness to at least explore an alternative. This phase is likely to involve several rounds of the tasks described, especially chair work with the EDP.

Moving on from Phase 2 does not require the tasks described to be fully worked through, rather the therapy will circle back to all of them in a 'two steps forward, one step back' means of progress (Pascual-Leone, 2018). As such, when Phase 2 has been sufficiently worked with, there is a notable (albeit tentative) curiosity or recognised need to look beyond the ED. There is a willingness to consider and hopefully some evidence of connection to emotion e.g. the ED Critic has deepened to a broader Critic and an (even vague) awareness of underlying vulnerability that can be explored. As such the client is no longer paralysed in stuckness and on some level has been able to access the Little Self, likely to reflect a move from secondary

Table 6.3 Stages in the ED Part Chair Work Task

Stage	Chair	Description of Task Stage	Useful Therapist Prompts
1. Identify the Marker & Initiate the Task – *Can we try something?*	Self chair	Client expresses symptom level distress caused by eating disorder thoughts and behaviours.	
2. Enact the EDP – *What Does the EDP Say?*	EDP chair	• Enact the EDP. • Be as specific and concrete as possible.	• Can you imagine yourself there and tell her some of what you were just saying?
3. Self Responds to the EDP – *What Does It Feel Like to hear the EDP Say Those Things?*	Self chair	• Elicit initial *emotional* reaction. • Deepen and Differentiate Self and EDP parts *(may require additional chair swops)*. • Identify core goals and messages of the EDP.	• What is it like to hear that, to be on the receiving end of that all day? • Clients who respond with agreement or thoughts should be directed back to how it *feels*.
4. Express the Unmet Need – *What Do You Need from the EDP Now?*	Self chair	• Express unmet need. • Support client in experiencing needs as valid.	• What do you need from her?
5. The EDP Responds to the Need – *Can the EDP Hear the Need?*	EDP chair	If EDP *shows (partial) compassion/ fear* – encourage its expression.	If EDP *shows no compassion* – name the rejection and enquire as to its function or its block.

(Continued)

Table 6.3 (Continued)

Stage	Chair	Description of Task Stage		Useful Therapist Prompts
6. Spark of the Healthy Adult – *Can the Power Differentials Begin to Shift?*	Self chair	**Negotiation & Integration** (If EDP showed compassion/ fear) – explore common goals and what small change might be possible.	**Setting Boundaries** (If EDP shows *no* compassion) – respond to the non-compassion, see if primary adaptive anger can be accessed.	**Setting Boundaries** – "How do you respond to her telling you, no, you must keep following her rules?" **Negotiation & Integration** – "What could this look like in practice? What would be possible?"
Debrief	Self chair	(a) Client reflects. (b) Therapist deeply validates any shifts/non-shifts and praises work done. (c) Make links back to the formulation. (d) Decide on appropriate action (e.g. homework).		

emotions of global distress/helplessness (reflective of coping modes) to core pain of shame of the self and of having needs.

References

Bowers, C., & Widdowson, M. (2023). Transactional analysis psychotherapy with clients who are neurodivergent: Experiences and practice recommendations. *International Journal of Transactional Analysis Research and Practice, 14*(1). 32–54. https://doi.org/10.29044/v14i1p32.

Brockmeyer, T., Holtforth, M. G., Bents, H., Kämmerer, A., Herzog, W., & Friederich, H.-C. (2012). Starvation and emotion regulation in anorexia nervosa. *Comprehensive Psychiatry, 53*(5), 496–501.

Denison-Day, J., Appleton, K. M., Newell, C., & Muir, S. (2018). Improving motivation to change amongst individuals with eating disorders: a systematic review. *International Journal of Eating Disorders, 51*(9), 1033–1050.

Dolhanty, J., & Greenberg, L. S. (2009). Emotion-focused therapy in a case of anorexia nervosa. *Clinical Psychology & Psychotherapy: An International Journal of Theory & Practice, 16*(4), 336–382.

Drinkwater, D., Holttum, S., Lavender, T., Startup, H., & Oldershaw, A. (2022). Seeing through the façade of anorexia: A grounded theory of emotional change processes associated with recovery from anorexia nervosa. *Frontiers in Psychiatry*, 13: 868586.

Elliott, R., Bohart, A., Larson, D., Muntigl, P., & Smoliak, O. (2023). Empathic reflections by themselves are not effective: Meta-analysis and qualitative synthesis. *Psychotherapy Research*, *33*(7), 957–973.

Elliott, R., & Greenberg, L. (2021). *Emotion-focused counselling in action*. Sage.

Elliott, R., Watson, J. C., Goldman, R. N., & Greenberg, L. S. (2004). *Learning emotion-focused therapy: The process-experiential approach to change*. American Psychological Association.

Elliott, R., Watson, J., Goldman, R.N., & Greenberg, L.S. (2025). *Learning emotion-focused therapy* (2nd ed.). APA.

Eun, B. (2019). The zone of proximal development as an overarching concept: A framework for synthesizing Vygotsky's theories. *Educational Philosophy and Theory*, *51*(1), 18–30.

Greenberg, L., Auszra, L., & Herrmann, I. (2007). The relationship among emotional productivity, emotional arousal and outcome in experiential therapy of depression. *Psychotherapy Research*, *17*(4), 482–493.

Greenberg, L. S. (2004). Emotion–focused therapy. *Clinical Psychology & Psychotherapy: An International Journal of Theory & Practice*, *11*(1), 3–16.

Greenberg, L. S. (2010). The Clinical Application of Emotion in Psychotherapy. In M. Lewis, J.M. Haviland-Jones, & L.F. Barrett, L. F. (Eds.), *Handbook of emotions* (pp. 88–101). Guilford Press.

Gregertsen, E. C., Mandy, W., & Serpell, L. (2017). The egosyntonic nature of anorexia: An impediment to recovery in anorexia nervosa treatment. *Frontiers in Psychology*, *8*, 2273.

Higbed, L., & Fox, J. R. (2010). Illness perceptions in anorexia nervosa: A qualitative investigation. *British Journal of Clinical Psychology*, *49*(3), 307–325.

Kinnaird, E., Stewart, C., & Tchanturia, K. (2019). Investigating alexithymia in autism: A systematic review and meta-analysis. *European Psychiatry*, *55*, 80–89.

Kyriacou, O., Easter, A., & Tchanturia, K. (2009). Comparing views of patients, parents, and clinicians on emotions in anorexia: A qualitative study. *Journal of Health Psychology*, *14*(7), 843–854.

Lesser, I. M. (1981). A review of the alexithymia concept. *Psychosomatic Medicine*, *43*(6), 531–543.

Loomes, R., & Bryant-Waugh, R. (2021). Widening the reach of family-based interventions for anorexia nervosa: Autism-adaptations for children and adolescents. *Journal of Eating Disorders*, *9*, 1–11.

Marco, E. J., Hinkley, L. B., Hill, S. S., & Nagarajan, S. S. (2011). Sensory processing in autism: A review of neurophysiologic findings. *Pediatric Research*, *69*(8), 48–54.

Martz, E., Weiner, L., Bonnefond, A., & Weibel, S. (2023). Disentangling racing thoughts from mind wandering in adult attention deficit hyperactivity disorder. *Frontiers in Psychology*, *14*, 1166602.

McKenzie, C., Rowley, L., Pugh, M., & Oldershaw, A. (2024). "It's literally like been life-changing": An Interpretative Phenomenological Analysis of a novel motivational chairwork intervention for the treatment of Anorexia Nervosa. *Authorea*. December 03, 2024. DOI: 10.22541/au.173320923.32150232/v1.

Muir, X., Preece, D. A., & Becerra, R. (2024). Alexithymia and eating disorder symptoms: the mediating role of emotion regulation. *Australian Psychologist*, *59*(2), 121–131.

Nimbley, E., Gillespie-Smith, K., Duffy, F., Maloney, E., Ballantyne, C., & Sharpe, H. (2023). "It's not about wanting to be thin or look small, it's about the way it feels": An IPA analysis of social and sensory differences in autistic and non-autistic individuals with anorexia and their parents. *Journal of Eating Disorders*, *11*(1), 89.

Noordenbos, G., Aliakbari, N., & Campbell, R. (2014). The relationship among critical inner voices, low self-esteem, and self-criticism in eating disorders. *Eating Disorders*, *22*(4), 337–351.

Oates, S. (2021). What if my "I'm ok, you're ok" is different from yours? Could the inherent optimism in transactional analysis be a form of compulsory ableism? *Transactional Analysis Journal*, *51*(1), 63–76.

Oldershaw, A., DeJong, H., Hambrook, D., Broadbent, H., Tchanturia, K., Treasure, J., & Schmidt, U. (2012). Emotional processing following recovery from anorexia nervosa. *European Eating Disorders Review*, *20*(6), 502–509.

Oldershaw, A., Startup, H., & Lavender, T. (2019). Anorexia nervosa and a lost emotional self: A psychological formulation of the development, maintenance, and treatment of anorexia nervosa. *Frontiers in Psychology*, *10*, 219.

Pascual-Leone, A. (2018). How clients "change emotion with emotion": A programme of research on emotional processing. *Psychotherapy Research*, *28*(2), 165–182.

Pérez Velázquez, J. L., & Galán, R. F. (2013). Information gain in the brain's resting state: A new perspective on autism. *Frontiers in Neuroinformatics*, *7*, 37.

Pettersen, G., Thune-Larsen, K. B., Wynn, R., & Rosenvinge, J. H. (2013). Eating disorders: challenges in the later phases of the recovery process: a qualitative study of patients' experiences. *Scandinavian Journal of Caring Sciences*, *27*(1), 92–98.

Prochaska, J. O., & DiClemente, C. C. (1983). Stages and processes of self-change of smoking: Toward an integrative model of change. *Journal of Consulting and Clinical Psychology*, *51*(3), 390.

Pugh, M., & Salter, C. (2018). Motivational chairwork: An experiential approach to resolving ambivalence. *European Journal of Counselling Theory, Research and Practice*, *2*, 1–15.

Rowley, L. (2023). *Motivation-enhancing interventions for people with eating disorders* Canterbury Christ Church University.

Samson, A. C., Huber, O., & Gross, J. J. (2012). Emotion regulation in Asperger's syndrome and high-functioning autism. *Emotion*, *12*(4), 659.

Saure, E., Raevuori, A., Laasonen, M., & Lepistö-Paisley, T. (2022). Emotion recognition, alexithymia, empathy, and emotion regulation in women with anorexia nervosa. *Eating and Weight Disorders-Studies on Anorexia, Bulimia and Obesity*, *27*(8), 3587–3597.

Schmidt, U., Startup, H., & Treasure, J. (2018). *A cognitive-interpersonal therapy workbook for treating anorexia nervosa: The Maudsley model*. Routledge.

Simpson, S., & Arntz, A. (2020). Core principles of imagery. In In G. Heath & H. Startup (Eds.), *Creative methods in schema therapy* (pp. 93–107). Routledge.

Startup, H., Lavender, A., Oldershaw, A., Stott, R., Tchanturia, K., Treasure, J., & Schmidt, U. (2013). Worry and rumination in anorexia nervosa. *Behavioural and Cognitive Psychotherapy*, *41*(3), 301–316.

Timulak, L., & Keogh, D. (2022). *Transdiagnostic emotion-focused therapy: A clinical guide for transforming emotional pain*. American Psychological Association.

Warwar, S. H., & Ellison, J. (2019). Emotion coaching in action: Experiential teaching, homework, and consolidating change. In L. S. Greenberg & R. N. Goldman (Eds.),

Clinical handbook of emotion-focused therapy (pp. 261–289). American Psychological Association. https://doi.org/10.1037/0000112-012.

Westwood, H., Kerr-Gaffney, J., Stahl, D., & Tchanturia, K. (2017). Alexithymia in eating disorders: Systematic review and meta-analyses of studies using the Toronto Alexithymia Scale. *Journal of Psychosomatic Research*, *99*, 66–81.

Williams, K., King, J., & Fox, J. R. (2016). Sense of self and anorexia nervosa: A grounded theory. *Psychology and Psychotherapy: Theory, Research and Practice*, *89*(2), 211–228.

Young, J. E., Klosko, J. S., & Weishaar, M. E. (2003). *Schema therapy: A practitioner's guide*. Guilford Press.

Chapter 7

Phase 3

Deepening to Core Pain

Having established a rationale and curiosity to work with emotion in Phase 2 (Chapter 6), as well as supporting clients to recognise links between symptom level distress and underlying emotional vulnerability, Phase 3, described in this chapter, supports clients to deepen their connection with emotion as they 'follow the pain'. This requires a degree of trust in the therapeutic relationship, such that emotion evoked can be sufficiently 'held' in the therapeutic space. Clients are likely to start to enter Phase 3 via work with the Eating Disorder Part (EDP) through which the broader Critic emerges (criticising characterological flaws). We begin this chapter by considering how to build on this and facilitate *deepening emotional experience* to access underlying stuck emotional processes. We describe linking this core pain and unmet need to episodic memories, grounding them within the developmental origins in which they emerged. This work to deepen the connection and understanding of core pain occurs in parallel to removing blocks to this process as they arise. Thus we continue to seek to *overcome avoidance of emotion,* and importantly, attention is paid to supporting *optimal emotion regulation* and bringing soothing for emotional vulnerability.

Deepening Connection with Emotional Experience

Phase 3 focuses on supporting clients to move past secondary emotions (and symptomatic processes) and bypass coping modes to become more aware of, regulate, and reflect on the core pain of the Little Self, predicated upon the basic principle that a person cannot leave a place until they have arrived there (Elliott & Greenberg, 2021). In Phase 2, the chair work task with the EDP can see the client and the EDP move through many phases. Gradually, the therapist can support the evolution of the EDP to uncover a broader critic underpinning the ED demands. This is achieved by encouraging greater specificity (e.g. "Tell her everything that will go wrong if she doesn't listen to you", "What will it mean for her if she doesn't listen to you?"). The EDP begins to reveal its primary motives, fear, and concerns such as "Everyone will reject you; People will see how worthless you are; You'll be a failure again." This reflects the painful emotion and internalised messages associated with shame (e.g. "You are broken/defective.") which can be deepened into

DOI: 10.4324/9781003468349-9

messages associated with lonely abandonment ("So if you show yourself to others they will reject you. You are unworthy of love and connection and are completely alone in life.") and gives way to the Little Self's expression of the needs aligned with these core painful primary feelings ("I needed to be heard/seen, to know I was worth something in your eyes, to feel your love and closeness."). This connection to core pain and unmet need is a necessary step in the emotional change processes underpinning SPEAKS, enabling us to work to transform these core painful feelings in Phase 4. Thus, 'Two-chair work for the Broader Inner Critic' deepens connection with emotional experience. This can be further elaborated by exploring its developmental origins in the 'Float Back' task.

Task: Two-chair Work for the Broader Inner Critic

As we encounter the broader Inner Critic we hear the historically based characterological or trait-like criticisms it proffers, leading to beliefs such as "I'm inferior, I'm worthless, I'm pathetic, I'm unlovable", which the client has sought to 'fix' or ameliorate via ED achievements and goals, alongside other forms of coping. The marker for this task is thus self-directed criticism. This may be explicit in the client narrative which the therapist can gently bring to their attention ("I hear that part of you that gives you a hard time, that is telling you again that you're stupid."). The inner critic may also get involved in the narrative brought during a task and in particular when working with the EDP. In the latter scenario, a therapist can choose whether to move the task on to working with the Inner Critic. This is quite easily and seamlessly achieved (by changing the EDP for the Inner Critic), and any opportunity to move to work with the Inner Critic should be seized, assuming there is the time within the session and willingness on the part of the client. Alternatively, recognition of the Inner Critic can be made and links back to formulation drawn, with this task bookmarked as a possible focus for a later session. This task is likely to evolve over time and deepen with each revisiting, it is likely clients will only get as far as differentiating from the critic in the first instance before deepening to the Little Self at a later time. In general the trajectory is that clients may move from a secondary emotional experience and coping modes, deepened into the Little Self and core pain, through to the primary adaptive emotion of the Healthy Adult.

Detailed Guidelines for the Inner Critic Task

Below are detailed guidelines on the 'Inner Critic' task and what may emerge or be required from the therapist in each step (adapted from Elliott & Greenberg, 2021; Elliott et al., 2004; Timulak & Keogh, 2020; summarised in Table 7.1).

Stage 1. Identifying the Marker and Initiating the Task – Can We Try Something?

The marker for this task is the presence of the Inner Critic within the session indicated by self-directed criticism, judgement, or contempt. The client may begin the session in this mode, or they may be observed to switch abruptly into this part of self, triggered by something during the session. It is likely that before you try this task you will have already brought the presence of the Critic gently to the client's attention and added it to the mode map. Criticisms can include judgements of behaviour or feelings, or be more globally directed at character or identity (e.g. "I'm stupid"; "I'm oversensitive"). Therapists carefully listen to the different types of criticisms or ways in which they can emerge, noting that they can also be projected onto an 'Other', which may need clarifying (e.g. "She thinks I'm an idiot." can be more accurately heard as "I think I am an idiot."). The therapist gently identifies the marker explicitly with the client. The language used can reflect that established in the mode map if appropriate.

- "I hear that part of you that is hard on yourself again. What is it that this part tells you about yourself? You're so ...?"
- "It would be really helpful to hear more about what happens there, when that critical part comes in, and how that affects you."

Stage 2. Enacting the Self-Criticism – *What Does the Critic Say?*

The therapist sets up a new chair facing opposite the client's current Self chair. The client is asked to move to the new chair (the Critic chair), to picture (or connect with a sense of) themselves in their original chair, and to enact the self-criticism: "Can you imagine yourself there and tell her some of what you were just saying? How you criticise her? You're such an idiot ..."

BE SPECIFIC AND AMPLIFY

The Critic is encouraged to be as specific and concrete as possible in their criticism, not just naming the criticism but the implications of that. For example, when the Critic says, "You let everybody down!" the therapist suggests, "Tell her all the ways she lets people down." or "Tell her what she 'should' have done; be specific."

The therapist pays attention to how the Critic speaks as well as what is said amplifying the tone and emotional expression: "I hear the disgust in what you are saying. Can you say it again and really show her your disgust?"

The purpose of enacting the criticism is not that we want to give the Critic airtime or are interested in adding any validity to their point of view, but rather to evoke and heighten emotion when the client moves back into the Self chair and also to better elicit its motivation and understand its protective or fearful position. To this end, criticisms which are related to perceived characterological flaws, vividly enacted, and with specificity are most useful here.

Note that, at the extreme, the Critic might reflect an annihilating self-critic (perhaps strongly connected to an abuser) that is extremely dysregulating and destabilising. If this emerges, chair work is suspended in favour of a more appropriate method of dealing with this self-destructive part of self. Appropriate tasks at this point include the 'Safe Bubble' exercise (see 'Optimising Emotion Regulation'), or even encouraging use of a coping mode to create a little distance. There may also need to be some graded exposure to a Critic that is especially harsh, hearing from this side for just a few moments at a time and learning to create distance such as using a metaphorical screen to create a little safety and respite.

> *Clara, It sounds like your Critic is especially harsh today, attacking you for having needs, as though it's actually dangerous to be human. This is a lot to bear. For a moment, close your eyes, and try to see if you can imagine that there is a moveable screen between Little Clara and your Critic, a screen that when you need a break you can just slide it across. See if you can have a go right now at creating that distance and space from your Critic.*

> *It may have been tough or even impossible to create distance when X (your parent, a bully) was attacking you, but as an adult, it's important to have choice about what messages we listen to. See how it feels gently using the moveable screen for a little break this week.*

Stage 3. Self Responds to the Criticism (Deepening to Core Pain of Little Self) – *What Does It Feel Like to Hear the Critic Say Those Things?*

Once the criticism has been clearly enacted and specified, the client returns to their original Self chair. When judging when to switch chairs, it can be useful to hold in mind the goals of each particular stage. Enacting and heightening the criticism (Stage 2) has the aim of evoking a deep emotional response when the client returns to the Self chair with the anticipation that the energy of the Critic will be matched in the level of emotional response. The goal in the Self chair (Stage 3) is to help the client differentiate from the Critic and deepen their emotion to the core pain of the Little Self. Indications that a switch back to the Self chair is desirable are:

- When the client starts to speak as if they are the Little Self, "It makes me feel so guilty when I don't …"
- When the client begins to show an emotional reaction in response to the Critic's words (e.g. they begin to cry) indicating an internal switch
- When the client expresses other changes in body language or facial expression suggesting an internal switch in reaction to the Critic's words (e.g. slumps in chair, looks defeated)

INITIAL EMOTIONAL REACTION TO THE CRITICISM

Once the client has returned to the Self chair, the therapist seeks to explore and encourages expression of emotion in response to the critical attack.

- "What does it feel like to hear that, Clara?"
- "What is it like for you to be on the receiving end of that?"

DEEPEN AND DIFFERENTIATE EMOTION TO ACCESS CORE PAIN OF
LITTLE SELF (INVOLVING CHAIR SWOPS BETWEEN CRITIC AND SELF, I.E.
STAGES 2 AND 3)

The therapist utilises their Emotion Coach approach with a gentle caring tone to probe for the Little Self and core pain. The client moves between inward attention to recognise and name feelings and then express them back to the critic if they can, explicating both the bodily feeling (e.g. shame) and associated action tendency (e.g. hide away). Empathic responding such as exploratory questions, conjecture and heightening can support the deepening process.

- "Can you look inside yourself, scan your body – your stomach, your chest, your face – and say what you feel in your body when you hear that?"

Going and back and forth between the Critic chair (Stage 2) and the Self chair (Stage 3) to support the differentiation of the parts, specificity of the Critic, and deepening of the client's experience facilitates accessing of core pain and connection with the Little Self. The specificity of the criticism and function of the Critic can be explored using prompts such as:

- "Tell her everything that will go wrong if she doesn't listen to you."
- "Tell her what her life will look like without you in it."
- "Tell her exactly why she needs you around."

This can be followed by reiterating the bottom-line message from the Inner Critic and an exploration of how the Inner Critic feels to say this, for example, "So tell her, I'm just trying to help. Because I'm what … worried about you … scared for you ….?"

Stage 4. Express the Unmet NEED – *What Does the Self Need from the Critic Now?*

Once the parts have been differentiated sufficiently and the client has connected with and expressed the core pain of the Little Self, they can be asked to consider what it is that they need from the Critic. The need we are seeking to articulate has a connection to the unmet needs of the Little Self, and therefore it is important that this part of self is sufficiently activated, otherwise it will not be clear or heartfelt in its expression. The client's ability to express the need can steer the therapist as to whether further deepening is required to access the core pain of Little Self (e.g. when a client says they don't know what they need). The nature of the need expressed can also point to a coping mode having emerged instead of the Little Self. For example, the Angry Protector who says, "I need you to get lost; I need you out of my life!" or the Helpless part who says, "There's no point even bothering, you'll never listen to me."

Where the Little Self has been sufficiently activated, the expression of the need reveals a deeper and more profound connection with the core pain. It initially often asks for a compromise, for a break or for the Critic to hear or trust in the Self more. This reflects shame-based core unmet needs for recognition, respect, and understanding (e.g. "I need you to hear me and trust me") and can be reflected back as such by the therapist. The act of asserting the need can itself generate an emotional shift in the client as they recognise and own the need, affording a sense of agency. This serves as a glimpse of the future Healthy Adult and the therapist should attune to such a shift and support its elaboration and expression. As this task is repeated, clients may be able to subsequently connect to the underlying core pain of lonely abandonment fears and sadness with unmet attachment needs (e.g. "I need to know and feel that you care"), a process more closely related to recovery from AN (Malik-Smith et al., in prep). Getting here to stage 4 reflects partial resolution of this task because there is a new emerging experience and narrative that the client can carry forward.

Stage 5. The Critic responds to the NEED – *Can the Critic Hear the Need?*

Once the client has connected with the Little Self, activated core pain, and expressed what they need, they return to the Critic chair and respond to this new expression of the Little Self. The therapist can direct the Critic to the key aspect of the need:

- "So Clara is saying, she is absolutely doing her best, is exhausted and you just keep making her feel worthless. She is asking for a break, at least sometimes, for you to not expect her to do so much."
- "How do you respond to this? Can you see her pain? How do you feel about her as she says this?"

Key to this stage is to assess whether the client can hear and respond to the core pain and unmet need. The response of the Critic is likely to reflect either rejection of the pain/needs and critical escalation, or compassion towards the pain/need (softening of the Critic).

THE CRITIC MAY *SHOW COMPASSION*

If the client as Critic expresses compassion towards the pain and unmet needs of the Self, the therapist seeks to deepen their expression of compassion to care, responsibility, remorse, and love amplifying any shifts in the view of the Little Self by the Critic.

- "How do you feel towards her?"
- "And how do you feel as you say this?"

Even where there is scope for the Critic to offer compassion, it can take several dialogues before this shift occurs, and this is indicative of the chronicity and tenacity of the self-judgement and self-critical processes (Timulak & Keogh, 2020). This is unsurprising given that the Critic will have had many years to develop and consolidate, and the client may hold onto a view of it being useful to them; therefore, loosening this process will take time. It is not uncommon for the Critic to show some compassion and partially soften in the face of the pain/need, but for this to be qualified in some way ("I had no idea it affected you like this. I can see now how hard it is for you, but also you need me. You'd be nothing without me").

THE CRITIC MAY *SHOW NO COMPASSION* AND REJECT NEEDS

In the case that the Critic shows no compassion and rejects the pain and needs expressed, therapists encourage the clear expression of that rejection. It is named and highlighted explicitly, followed by an enquiry around what blocks compassion and/or the function of rejection.

- "Tell Clara: I don't care how you feel. I am going to continue pushing you."
- "What drives you to reject what she tells you she feels and needs?"
- "What would happen if she didn't have you pushing her?"

Asking these questions can reveal the protective nature of the Critic and highlighting this affords the client opportunity to respond to the function (in Stage 6), rather than to the harsh judgement and self-attack.

Stage 6. Foundations of the Healthy Adult – *Can Feelings of the Healthy Adult Be Experienced and Expressed (Acceptance or Assertive Anger)?*

Now the client to moves back to the Self chair, and we see if core pain can begin to be transformed by accessing primary adaptive emotions (e.g. compassion, assertive anger, grief), which are the foundations of the Healthy Adult. Thus, it is in this stage that we might see the client start to tentatively shift from Little Self to Healthy Adult who can be (newly) experienced with a sense of self-agency, with this shift becoming more evident over time with repetition of the task and especially after greater transformation work in Phase 4.

ACCEPTANCE (IF CRITIC *SHOWS COMPASSION*)

If the Critic has been able to express a compassionate response, when the client moves back to the Self chair, we want them to truly experience and take in that compassion.

- "How does it feel to hear the critical part say she is sorry, she had no idea it had had this affect on you, and that she will try to give you space and let you do it on your terms?"
- "Can you let that in?"
- "What happens inside when you hear that response –I hear you and I do care …?"
- "How do you see this critical part now?"

Therefore, the process of letting in compassion involves both noticing and hearing the compassion and also reflecting on what it feels like to receive that compassion. These feelings can include primary adaptive emotions reflecting the soothing nature of the compassion, such as relief or acceptance. The therapist also listens for any shifts in the view of the critic, such as being less powerful or a reciprocated compassion. By truly connecting with the compassion and the felt sense of that the client can shift in their self-organisation, taking in the self-supportive processes of the Healthy Adult and shifting the relationship with the Critic.

ASSERTIVE ANGER (IF CRITIC *SHOWS NO COMPASSION*)

If the Critic has not shown compassion or has escalated in their criticism in response to expression of need, the client can instead be encouraged to build a sense of assertive anger, which is also a self-supportive Healthy Adult process. Their response to the lack of compassion is explored. Note that here we are encouraging the client to move to the Healthy Adult rather than access further the pain of the Little Self. As such, in this case, the therapist does not ask the client to look inside at how it feels to have received no compassion, but rather encourages them to respond, assessing the client's ability to assert themselves.

- "How do you respond to her treating you this way?"
- "Is this ok with you?"

The client can also be encouraged to react to the protective function of the critic, if one has been established.

"You say you are trying to help me, but you just get in my way, you stop me from doing the things I enjoy."

Here the freshly emerging Healthy Adult and the Critic can negotiate and newly integrate. By moving back and forth between Critic and Healthy Adult chairs, a more unified perspective can be established.

Debrief

Once the task is finished, reflecting on the resolution or where the task has reached before the session ends is an important part of the process.

(a) **Client reflects.** Client reflects on what they notice from the task trying to tease out any meaning made. What do they take away? Ask the client to put into a first person 'I' statement (e.g. I deserve to try something new; I don't deserve to be spoken to like that, I have done nothing wrong; I feel a sense of relief; I feel stronger).

(b) **Therapist deeply validates any shifts/non-shifts, praises work done and prizes emotion shared.** The therapist can reflect newly identified core messages back to the client: "It is so moving to hear you say you deserve more, you really do, and I'd love to see how knowing this can make a difference for you."

(c) **Make links back to the formulation.** Clearly connect what has emerged to the part map. Reflect on any patterns between parts that were newly observed during the chair task and add to the map if appropriate/significant. Core painful emotions and associated unmet needs can be added to a client's part map as part of the Little Self to further support understanding and conceptualisation of these. Highlight where the new experiences indicate change has occurred or might be needed as a focus of future work.

(d) **Decide on any appropriate action, ideas of different experiences or actions that might be tried between sessions.** Try to keep this collaborative and client directed. Homework that incorporates greater awareness is valuable. Asking clients to listen out for the emergence of the Critic in their week and notice how they respond when it emerges can be valuable task between sessions. They can experiment with gaining a little distance from the Critic, such as imagining the movable screen, a safe bubble or to turning a 'volume' dial to quieten it down.

Additional Considerations, Including for Neurodivergent Clients

Setting Up the Task

As with all tasks, the therapist seeks the client's agreement for the task and collaboratively sets it up, emphasising there are no expectations. As highlighted in previous chapters, autistic clients may have a tendency to think concretely and literally so attention should be paid to ensuring that the client understands the purpose of the task and has space to ask any questions before completing it for the first time. Undoubtedly this can feel like a strange task, although it is likely that some chair work with the EDP will have been completed at this stage. Normalising this and supporting the client to move beyond hesitancy or inauthenticity can help to allow themselves into the task. Letting the client know that there are no 'right' answers, there is no expected script that you are hoping they will follow, but treating all tasks as an exploration of client process can reassure some concerns.

Some clients may not be able to visually 'picture' themselves in the other chair (e.g. aphantasia), and for others, visualisation can feel odd and distracting or take all attentional resources. Guiding clients to gain a 'sense' of the other can be more beneficial. In general, having therapists be curious of how clients explore their internal world during the mode mapping phase, and their most prominent senses, can afford insights into how to maximise chair work. Using the object chosen during mode mapping to represent a part of self within a chair or using a photograph (e.g. of Current or Little Self) can be a prompt to bring parts, emotions and thoughts to life if needed.

Staying Attuned

It is possible that a client will move back into the EDP following a focus on the broader Inner Critic, commenting on physical flaws or ED behaviours. Here the therapist can support the client to access the broader Critic again by asking the EDP to be specific about what it means for the client to gain weight or to change body shape and what it will say about them if they do. If the client keeps moving back to the EDP, switching to chair work with the EDP may be necessary, and this task will need to be revisited later. Throughout, the therapist remains empathically attuned, guiding the process of client in dialogue with the Critic utilising the focusing inwards process, using heightening responses, empathic conjecture, mirroring client language, and bringing emphasis to poignant feelings ("Say that again, it makes me feel …") to support emotion expression with specificity. If the client is able to non-verbally express emotion but is struggling to bring meaning or narrative to that, encourage them to verbalise their experiences (e.g. "Can you speak from the tears?") or be more specific about the physical sensations ("What does that tightening in your chest say?"). Therapist's tone and their emotional expression in empathic responses are especially important to facilitate emotional deepening and in welcoming, holding and gently affirming painful emotion. Without this support, autistic clients may otherwise find it difficult to answer questions about emotions (Loomes & Bryant-Waugh, 2021).

Attuning to the client's style and speed of emotion process and expression is needed. People with anorexia and neurodivergent people can vary widely in their emotional expression; for example, having a flat tone or facial expression that can obscure emotion felt or use restricted language even for emotion that is evidently present. The therapist can tentatively and curiously name and express what they see or feel that is still on edges of awareness. Dialogical contact with the therapist is kept to a minimum, although the therapist remains closely connected and can be used as a resource for emotion regulation (see 'Emotion Coaching', Chapter 6).

Neurodivergent people in particular may experience sensory differences and, as such, may be processing a wider array of sensory experiences in any one moment.

Alongside other interoceptive differences, this can make the process for clients to home in on the experience and expression of a felt emotional sense a slow one. Patience and gentle exploration is required on the part of therapist. Explicitly guiding the client into their body, being curious about what and where sensory experiences are located can be followed with empathic conjectures to connect sensations to feelings words. This can also be a support for clients who are alexithymic. You will know your client well by now and what their specific needs are, but additional small adjustments such as asking them to close their eyes to better focus on interoceptive sensory information with fewer distractions can be useful in guiding the deepening process.

Lack of Differentiation from and/or Agreement with the Critic

Clients can struggle to differentiate from the Critic, especially when it is newly introduced. Those critical messages have been such an embedded part of the client's experience that it can be hard to separate from them and begin to look on at them; the Self and Critic are very enmeshed. For this reason, clients may initially spontaneously use critical statements even when sitting in the Self chair, especially before they have sufficiently deepened into the core pain of the Little Self. It can take a few repetitions of this task for a client to tease them apart and more consistently experience the parts as separate. Therapists listen out for the Critic popping up and can ask the client to switch back to the Critic chair when it emerges and repeat the same critical statement from there, so that each side is clear and owns its experience. The client is always encouraged to use 'You' statements in the Critic chair (to reflect the blaming quality) and 'I' statements in the 'Self' chair (to reflect the received impact).

Another very common part of the process is for a client to agree with the Critic ("She's right; I'm pathetic and stupid"). This can be acknowledged and validated by the therapist ("So you agree with her."), but it reflects the secondary emotions of a helpless and surrendering coping mode; therefore we want to move past that and not get stuck in this aspect of the dialogue. To achieve this, the client requires redirecting to the painful feelings evoked by such attacks ("But what do you feel as you hear her say this?"). Therapist then continues to explore the client's internal experience and the expression of that to the Critic to access freshly experienced core pain. If the client continues to find accessing emotion difficult or focuses on agreement with the Critic, the client can return to the Critic chair and the criticism is again heightened to evoke fresh emotion upon return to the Self chair. This process may need some patient repeating and holding to enable clients to deepen to the core pain and access the Little Self.

Flipping to a Coping Mode

It can be common for the client, upon returning to the Self chair, to respond to the Critic from a coping mode. After all, this is their hypothesised usual internal process – to move to a coping mode following a critical attack that has triggered the core pain of the Little Self. Clients placate the Critic and its demands (e.g. an overcompensatory part) in order to gain acceptance (from the Critic and people at the heart of its developmental origins), respond by self-protecting with the rejecting anger of the Angry Protector ("I won't listen to this; I hate you."), surrender into agreement with the Critic, or just avoid the pain that is triggered (e.g. Detached Protector). In such a case, the therapist must decide whether to continue with this task or to move into two-chair work with this self-interruption (see 'Overcoming Avoidance of Emotion' in this chapter). Just acknowledging the emotional response, perhaps to name the part of self and notice that it is getting in the way here, can shift this block sufficiently to complete the task at hand. For clients with better visual memory or who are visual thinkers, this can be visually supported. For example, the client could retrieve the formulation object for this interrupting coping mode and physically put it to one side, placing it as far away as they feel they can have it at this moment or facing the opposite direction.

Supporting the Healthy Adult

Clients may access the adaptive emotions of the Healthy Adult weakly and with variability, moving between assertive anger and standing up to the Critic and then being unable to. In this case the therapist responds with empathy, acknowledging and empathising with how hard it can be to stand up to the Critic, whilst hoping to maintain connection with the Healthy Adult. This connection can be achieved by highlighting the Critic's mistreatment of the client. Likewise, being evocative in amplifying the depths of the client's inability to respond can also facilitate pushback in the form of assertive anger.

- "Tell her, I can't stand up to you; you're too strong."
- "Tell her I will blindly follow your rules to the letter" If the client sees this is a step too far and will not say it: "So tell her, I am not going to just blindly follow your rules and whatever you say any more. I want to be guided by my own needs."

Task: Float Back for Accessing Episodic Memories to Connect to Core Pain

Core painful feelings such as those accessed during the Inner Critic task are not new nor unknown feelings for our clients. They can be described as a 'bad, stuck old feelings' (Greenberg & Elliott, 2012) which, as described, clients commonly go to some lengths to avoid. It is argued that this core pain was first encountered in developmental experiences relating to chronic unmet needs. Subsequent relationships and situations, including in the present day, which resonate with this feeling and associated unmet needs easily trigger associated schema beliefs (such as "I am 'unlovable' and destined for 'abandonment.'") along with the full force of the associated core pain (Simpson & Arntz, 2020; Timulak & Keogh, 2020). Connecting episodic

Table 7.1 Stages in the Two-chair Task for the Broader Inner Critic

Stage	Chair	Description of Chair Work Inner Critic Task Stage	Useful Therapist Prompts
Stage 1. Identify the Marker & Initiate the Task – *Can We Try Something?*	Self chair	Client expresses harsh, critical self-judgement, self-contempt, or self-treatment.	
Stage 2. Enact the Critic – *What Does the Critic Say?*	Critic chair	• Enact the self-criticism. • Be specific (about the criticism and why it is needed). • Amplify critic tone and expression.	• "I hear that part of you that is hard on yourself again. What is it that this part tells you about yourself? You're so ...?" • "How does it feel, when you talk to yourself like this?"
Stage 3. Self Responds to the Critic – *What Does It Feel Like to Hear the Critic Say Those Things?*	Self chair	• Elicit initial *emotional* reaction. • Deepen and differentiate Self and Critic parts *(may require additional chair swops)*. • Deepen to access core pain of Little Self. • Express core pain to Critic.	• "What does it feel like to hear that? 'You're pathetic.'" • "What is it like for you (Little Self) to be on the receiving end of that?"
Stage 4. Self expresses the unmet Need – *What Does the Self Need from the Critic now?*	Self chair	• Self expresses unmet need *(where the emotions have been sufficiently deepened this reflects the core pain and unmet needs of the Little Self).* • Listen for further emotional shifts.	• Can you (Little Self) tell her what you need?
Stage 5. The Critic Responds to the Need – *Can the Critic Hear the Need?*	Critic chair	If critic **shows compassion** – encourage its expression and how it feels to express compassion. If critic shows **no compassion** – heighten the rejection.	• "How do you respond to this? Can you see her pain? How do you feel about her as she tells you this?"

Table 7.1 (Continued)

Stage	Chair	Description of Chair Work Inner Critic Task Stage		Useful Therapist Prompts
Stage 6. Healthy Adult Emerges – *Can the Feelings of the Healthy Adult be Experienced and Expressed?*	Self chair	**Acceptance** (If critic *showed* compassion) – let it in and reflect what it feels like to receive it and what it means for the client now	**Assertive Anger** (If critic *shows no* compassion) – respond to the non-compassion, see if primary adaptive anger can be accessed	**Acceptance –** "Can you let that in? What happens inside?" **Assertive Anger –** "How do you respond to her treating you this way? Is this ok with you?"
Debrief	Self chair	(a) Client reflects (b) Therapist deeply validates any shifts/non-shifts and praises work done (c) Make links back to the formulation (d) Decide on appropriate action (e.g. homework)		

memories to core pain and unmet need opens up opportunities for further processing and change. Clients may easily identify and name memories in which this feeling resonates. Often those first recalled pertain to recent relationships, e.g. partner/friend/ bully. There may, however, be times when clients need support to access memories of core pain or when the narrative retelling does not sufficiently afford an emotional connection. Indeed, imagery evokes more emotion than verbal processing of the same material (Holmes et al., 2007). This may be particularly true in relation to accessing core painful feelings in memories of developmental relationships. For clients who find it hard to experientially access emotion, imaginal exposure to earlier memories can usefully deepen, evoke and heighten emotion. It can also bring more clarity around the reasons for and origins of an emotional reaction.

Imaginal exposure to past memories is used in both Schema Therapy (ST; Simpson & Arntz, 2020) and Emotion Focused Therapy (EFT; Greenberg, 2021). The 'Float Back' task from ST in particular offers a helpful guide to support clients in using memory to connect with core pain and unmet need (Simpson & Arntz, 2020). To engage in this task clients need a sufficient degree of Healthy Adult to draw on to help 'hold onto' the experience of a memory being worked with, rather than being back in the past. It is important that the client does not simply 'regress' or disappear into a split off traumatised child part – reaching a regressed state is not the goal of this type of imagery work and is usually a sign that connection with the therapist or Healthy Adult is lost. If a client gets lost within the memory as though they are right back there, then this is likely to be a flashback indicating little or no contact with the Healthy Adult. Rather, clients are guided to contact a significant memory to the degree that it is within their 'reach' (i.e. they fall upon it with relative ease) and task enquiry about the needs of the child within the memory and so a degree of 'meta-perspective' is maintained. Where clients have endured significant early life trauma that has not been processed at a narrative and cognitive level then working with early developmental memories and images in this way is not indicated until later in the therapy process and when suitable resources have been established.

This work has a range of functions: facilitating access to painful emotions, elucidating the origins of a current schematic and emotional reaction to inform formulation and enabling validation of emotions in the context they first occurred. Later in Phase 4, the 'Float Back' task incorporates a rescripting of the past origin scene in any way needed so as to create new emotional connections, a change in imagery as well as in schematic meaning (Simpson & Arntz, 2020). This task may be repeated many times throughout therapy, sometimes linked to the same cluster of schema and unmet needs so that optimal processing of associated emotion and cognitive learning takes place.

Detailed Guidelines for Float Back Task

Stage 1. Identifying the Marker and Initiating the Task – Can We Try Something?

The marker for this task is when a client presents with an experience of core pain (in the current session or from between sessions) and they are ready to further connect with it and explore its original themes. Clients will have an elaborated narrative of their early life and be sufficiently resourced to regulate affect that comes with access to early life painful memories before attempting this task (see Table 7.2).

Stage 2. Evoke and Elaborate the Association or Memory – Tell Me More about When This Feeling Came

IDENTIFY A PRESENT-DAY TRIGGER FOR CORE PAIN

First the goal is to evoke the core pain in the session if it is not present. The most 'live' way of doing this is to invite the client to think of a time in the recent past when they felt connection with this emotional state, even fleetingly. The client is then invited to sit comfortably with their eyes closed (or fixed on a spot in the room) and asked to unfold the scene (prompting them to remain in the first person when retelling).

With your eyes closed and in the first person, try to recall a recent time when you felt in touch with that feeling of shame [pause and give them a moment].

Now, in your mind's eye, like a scene playing out right now, please walk though and describe the events that lead up to that flood of emotion. When you are in contact with the flood of feeling, I may guide you a little.

Stage 3. Connect with and Deepen the Core Pain – *Can We Make This Feeling 'Bigger'?*

As the client reaches the point of emotional activation in their description of the experience (the 'hot' moment when the emotion was at its strongest), the therapist's goal is to help them to make this feeling as present as possible, to support their embodied connection with it.

FOCUS INWARDS

Therapist uses their stance as emotion coach to encourage the client to focus inwards as a means to connect with their emotional experience and supports the 'felt sense' of the emotion.

- "Now I know this is tough, but I'd like you to stay with these difficult feelings of shame, and can you tell me where in your body these feelings are located: your tummy? Your chest? Your head?"
- "How would you describe the way you feel right now?"
- "Are there any thoughts racing through your head?"
- "Is there anything you feel yourself doing in response to this feeling?"

MAKE THE FEELINGS 'BIG' TO DEEPEN CONNECTION

When the client is in touch with the full spectrum of senses associated with the feelings, the goal is to support them in deepening these feelings.

Now I try to make these feelings as big as possible, let them fill your body, really let them grow, can you feel them in your chest/tummy/legs? I know this is hard work, but try to let them in, let them fill your body.

The therapist can use their attuned empathic stance to assess the level of client's connection with emotion as well as non-verbal indications that they are fully in touch with the feeling, e.g. facial expressions, tears in the eye, a subdued or submissive body posture.

Stage 4. Float Back – *Is There an Earlier Memory That Fits with This Feeling?*

Stage 4 involves attempting to locate earlier memories with the same emotional tone as the current memory.

HOLD ON TO THE FEELING AND CLEAR THE MIND OF CURRENT MEMORY

The therapist asks the client to stay with this feeling but to clear the images and experiences linked to the current memory.

> *Now I want you to stay with these feelings but to erase the present images of this memory from your mind, the one with xxxxx, just let that go. But please stay with this deep and painful shame.*

FIND AN EARLIER MEMORY WITH THIS SAME FEELING

Next the therapist seeks to form an 'affect bridge' guiding the client to access an earlier memory or association linked to this feeling state. The goal is to help them go back as far as they can to an early, often relational memory or significant encounter.

> *Let your mind wander backwards to a time earlier in your life when these same feelings were present. Try to find an earlier memory or state with these same or similar feelings attached.*

The therapist should give the client time and space to drift back with these feelings. It may be that the first time this task is completed the earliest memories, those rooted in developmental relationships are not accessed because interruptions or blocks to memory or feeling emerge (e.g. a detached mode or Critic), evident in the client being distracted or beginning to distance themselves.

Stage 5. Elaborate the Memory or Association – *Tell Me More about the New Memory of This Feeling*

GET A DETAILED DESCRIPTION OF THE NEW MEMORY ACCESSED

Once your client is ready, and has fallen upon an associated memory or image, gently ask for details and spend time elaborating the scene so that you both fully and dynamically appreciate it.

> *Who is there?*
> *How old are you?*
> *What is happening?*
> *Who is involved?*
> *What are you feeling?*
> *What is the worst bit of it/most painful part?*
> *What did the Little You need in the image?*

The goal is to understand the unmet needs of the client in the image and the contribution of early relationships and events. Whilst it is valuable to gather a general sense of the contributing relationships and situations, the worst part of the memory should not be explored in detail. In fact, the therapist should pause the image before any trauma takes place. If trauma memories are accessed, the task is paused, and suitable grounding techniques are employed to stabilise and reorient the client to the present moment.

Debrief

Invite the client to open their eyes and re-orient them to the room. Debrief by asking the client to reflect on the experience of the float back:

(a) **Client reflects.** Ask the client what it was like linking back to the earlier scene, what do they make of the link between the present-day trigger and past scene? What have we learned about their early relationships and unmet need?
(b) **Therapist deeply validates any shifts/non-shifts and stays with emotion shared.** The client can be directed towards self-soothing at the end of the session and for between sessions (see 'Working for Optimal Emotion Regulation', this chapter).
(c) **Make links back to the formulation.** Clearly connect what has emerged to the part map and highlight where the new experiences indicate change has occurred or might be needed as a focus of future work (such as how unmet need links to core pain)
(d) **Decide on any appropriate action, ideas of different experiences or actions that might be tried between sessions.** Try to keep this collaborative and client directed. For this task it could be to 'check in' with their Experiencing Self daily so they feel 'heard' and 'seen' and any of the core pains of the earlier scene are not repeated.

Clara

Clara had been triggered by an experience at work where she had been giving a presentation and had been corrected on a minor point by her boss in front of a room full of her peers. She had been continually ruminating on it ever since. Exploring the emotion, she described feeling hot and shrinking into herself, eventually naming the experience as overwhelming shame. Using the 'Float Back' Clara fell upon a memory of being in the school dinner hall around age nine. She had spilt her drink all over her plate of food, but she was refused a replacement serving and told she had to eat what she was already given. As Clara ate it, she felt disgusted with the meal. She forced the food down as her cheeks burned with shame while her peers looked on giggling and whispering to each other. Clara said that she had needed someone to offer her understanding and to tell her they knew it wasn't her fault (reflecting unmet identity needs). As she stayed with the image, Clara began to notice how completely alone and rejected she had felt in that moment with nobody to turn to (reflecting unmet attachment needs), and that that was the most painful part; her feelings moved to include a deep sadness.

As these painful feelings came in, Clara's therapist noticed Clara wrap her arms around herself. Her therapist guided Clara's attention to this containing sensation and encouraged her to experiment to find the right amount of pressure to feel calmer and safe. At the end of the session, they discussed ways Clara would look after herself this week and how she might continue this soothing action. In line with her 'limited reparenting' stance to meet the unmet need expressed, her therapist sent Clara an email two days later to maintain their connection, to let her know she was there in the background and was thinking of her.

Additional Considerations, Including for Neurodivergent Clients

The following considerations apply to both this initial Float Back task and the Float Back with Rescripting introduced in Phase 4.

Lack of an Image/Memory or One That Is Very Vague

As described throughout this guidebook, attuning to a client's preferred processing style and differences is important; thus, symbolising in words, images, and/or actions can be utilised as appropriate. Furthermore, it may be that for the first few times the client's Detached Protector comes in and diverts the task. If this is the case, it can be useful to name this part and gently ask this mode to step aside:

I know you are only trying to help Clara because she probably feels a bit scared right now but other parts of her really want to learn to feel more. Please, Detached Protector, can you step aside and perhaps go wait at the door (there for when Clara leaves) and let Clara come back to the feelings she is trying to get alongside.

Difficulty Identifying Unmet Needs in the Image

If a client is very young in the image (younger than six years) then it is best not to ask them what they need. Few six-year-olds can answer this question! Here, the style is for the therapist to use their reparenting skills and empathy and sensitively enquire about the needs of the young child:

You are all alone and only five years old. That is not ok. How about I come into the image, or someone else you feel safe with comes in, and you can tell us where you want us to stand so that you feel safe and cared for and there are adults alongside you.

Dismissing the Value of this Type of Task

A client may say, "Well, it wasn't like that for me as a child, so what's the point of this?" This points towards further work in Phase 4 to work with acknowledging and grieving the loss of unmet need setting up a useful opportunity to deepen the next phase of work in the direction of emotional processing of anger, sadness, regret and loss. Therapists empathically acknowledge that we cannot change the past and this can make it a bitter-sweet experience to get in touch with how things 'should' have been.

Ensuring Safety before Ending

In Phase 3, the task explores memories with a goal for these feelings to be heard and validated and for unmet needs to be illuminated. Later in Phase 4, a rescripting step is introduced with the goal being for the client to have their needs met to a limited degree, e.g. they should feel somewhat safer, seen, cared for, or protected. If the memory they are with is one of significant harm, then the image ends when the threat is no longer present and the child reports feeling safe. It is also important to check out secondary worries, such as a bully returning to 'get them back' once the therapist has left and address this before leaving the image (e.g. shrink the bully down into a small creature, or have the child leave the school altogether never to return). You can use scaling questions to regularly check in with a client as to whether the need has been achieved sufficiently. A useful time to close the image is when the client's needs have been sufficiently validated or (if rescripting) to have been met to a degree that are observably calmer in their body and you can notice a feeling shift. A useful question to ask yourself as therapist would be, if this was an actual child, would it feel right to leave them at this point? Or does more need to be done? It can also be useful to ask the client: What needs to happen for you to feel even safer?

Inability to Connect with or Animosity towards the Little Self

Prior to any task with the younger self the client will need to have accessed some warmth towards their younger self and done so with vulnerability and need. Where this is a struggle in imagery or the client flounders, the therapist can seek permission to enter the image and support this, supporting both the further experience of the Healthy Adult and self-compassion (see Phase 4 for 'Float Back with Rescripting' for further detail on this approach).

> *You are just a little girl and I can see such sadness on your face, can you let me come into the image offer her something, a teddy maybe. Perhaps you and I [the therapist] sit alongside her, and we can remind her that we are here for her and she is not alone. No young child should be all alone like this.*

Overcoming Avoidance of Emotion

Chronic core pain hurts when attended to, and clients have understandably developed ways to manage and avoid such feelings, as well as taking measures to avoid the generation of new feelings (e.g. by avoiding conflict with others), using coping modes (e.g. people-pleasing to placate others even where it means suppressing one's

Table 7.2 Stages in the Float Back Task

Stage	Description of Float Back Stage	Key Therapist Responses
Stage 1. Identify the Marker & Initiate the Task – *Can We Try Something?*	Client recalls memories of relationships which feel traumatic due to core pain attached or a specific incident which has happened recently where core pain was triggered.	
Stage 2. Elaborate Details of the Memory – *Tell Me More about when This Feeling Came*	• Describe the memory in detail.	- With your eyes closed and in the first person, try to recall a recent time when you felt in touch with that same feeling. - Please walk though and describe the events that led up to that flood of emotion.
Stage 3. Connect with and Deepen the Feeling – *Can We Make This Feeling 'Bigger'?*	• Focus inwards. • Support the 'felt sense' of the emotion. • Make the feeling 'big' to deepen connection.	- Tell me where in your body these feelings are located: your tummy? Your chest? Your head? How would you describe the way you feel right now?
Stage 4. Roll Back – *Is There an Earlier Memory That Fits with This Feeling?*	• Hold on to the feeling and clear mind of current memory • Find an earlier memory with this same feeling.	- Stay with these feelings but erase the present memory from your mind. - Try to find an earlier memory or state with these same feelings attached.
Stage 5. Elaborate the Memory or Association – *Tell Me More about the Earlier Memory of this Feeling*	• Get a detailed description of the new memory accessed. • Get a description of the client, including age in the memory, and who else was present.	Please can you describe to me the scene before you? Who is there? What is happening? What is the worst bit of it/ most painful part? What did you need in the image?
Debrief	(a) Client reflects. (b) Therapist deeply validates any shifts/ non-shifts and praises work done. (c) Make links back to the formulation. (d) Decide on appropriate action (e.g. homework).	

own needs), and symptomatic behaviours, such as excessive exercise, focusing on calories and weight, or binging. Through formulation of a client's mode map, they will by now have developed a better understanding of how parts developed, their patterns of coping and how/when this becomes unhelpful. The focus of Phase 3 on connecting with core pain will be difficult for clients and trigger interruptions to connecting with the Little Self in the above tasks, hindering a client's ability to process painful feelings and identify unmet needs. Coping modes commonly emerge as blocks to other tasks, observed as the client engages in dialogue at a superficial level such as falling into overcompensating, surrendering or rejecting of parts.

A goal of Phase 3 is to continue to work directly with emotion avoidance processes as they emerge. This is often achieved in the emotional attunement and 'limited reparenting' stance of the therapist who acknowledges and validates secondary emotions but seeks to move past them to focus on core pain and the Little Self. The therapist empathically guides a client back to bypassed emotions and to stay with them such as by using evocative reflections (heightening emotional language using imagery: "It's like this void opens up inside you."), empathic affirmations (witnessing and holding the pain when it comes: "I see how much this hurts."), empathic refocusing (guiding clients back to bypassed emotion: "So yes, you just walked away, but there was this real anger there in that moment..."), and focusing on their embodied experience ("How does it feel inside as you talk about this now?").

Understanding of the function and development of coping modes will have been explored in Phase 1 when developing the mode map, therefore conceptualisation about the role of a coping mode and the purpose of its current emergence in this moment can be reflected upon. Highlighting (as opposed to working to directly challenge) the process can be sufficient to bypass such parts and remove them as a block to accessing core pain whilst maintaining the focus of the original task. Some coping modes will almost always emerge at least early in therapy and the presence of a coping mode should not always be considered indicative of a sufficiently strong marker for directly working with them, however, coping modes that are persistently obstructive to accessing core pain can be addressed using 'Two-chair Work with Coping Modes' task.

Task: Two-chair Work with Coping Modes

Where clients are too 'stuck' within coping modes to move to deeper work or these interruptions/blocks are too strongly interfering they can be worked with in a specific and detailed way. This can be done using a two-chair task to facilitate dialogue with the coping mode. In ST, sometimes multiple chairs are used to work with coping modes and these adaptations are described elsewhere (Heath & Startup, 2020).

As with all tasks, this chair work task follows a step process to resolution, with the goal of reducing the impact of the coping mode on the client. The pattern of this task using chairs is similar to the chair work task used with the EDP (Phase 2, chapter 6) and the Inner Critic (Phase 3, this chapter) (Elliott & Greenberg, 2021). There are differences in the goals and modes that can emerge in response however. The key difference is that, in chair work with the Critic, we hear from the Critic to evoke emotion in the Self and support deepening to the core pain and unmet needs of the Little Self, allowing for adaptive emotions to emerge and begin building the Healthy Adult. In the chair dialogue with the coping modes, we want to hear from the coping modes to learn more about their behaviours, functions and fears (what will happen if they are not there). This can include the self-neglect of surrendering modes, self-interruption of avoiding modes, and self-coercion of overcompensating modes. Here it also has some parallels with the interviewing and exploring of modes described in mode mapping (Phase 1, Chapter 5). This chair task puts the self and the coping mode into direct dialogue enabling deeper exploration of the *emotional* impact of this way of coping to access adaptive emotions of the Healthy Adult and begin negotiate to set limits with the coping mode leading to more favourable reintegration. In contrast to the Critic chair work, the Healthy Adult is not usually accessed via the Little Self here. The 'Two-chair Work with Coping Modes' task is described in Table 7.3.

Clara

Clara struggled with a Detached Protector part that interrupted and blocked her feelings. Although she had begun to be able to feel and access emotion, following the 'Float Back' task, this part had become very strong, blocking her progress in therapy. Her therapist validated this understandable shift after accessing painful feelings, which went some way to help, but when Clara came to therapy the next week still feeling extremely detached, they agreed that directly exploring this part and how it was affecting her would be useful. Clara's 'gorilla' Detached Protector told her that feeling things ended badly, it was too painful to bear, and she would become overwhelmed and unable to cope if she continued allowing herself to feel, reflecting unhelpful beliefs about emotions.

Clara (as coping mode):	*If you allow yourself to feel this you won't be able to stop, you're never able to manage your feelings, you'll just feel dreadful forever.*
Therapist:	*So you are trying to help? To protect her? To make sure she copes?*
Clara:	*Yes, exactly. She needs me. [Then to Self chair] You need me. You wouldn't cope without me.*
Therapist:	*Because what will go wrong if she allows her feelings to come?*
Clara:	*Other people will notice and they'll know how weak and pathetic you are. They'll be judging you. I am protecting you from that. From other people rejecting you. I help you hide yourself.*
Therapist:	*So it's not just that expressing emotion makes you weak …. it's that it's actually dangerous … it makes you vulnerable and at risk of getting hurt.*
Clara:	*Yes.*
Therapist:	*So, this is what you do to yourself instead. Hide yourself away.*

Clara moves to Self chair

Therapist:	*What's it like when that part of you shuts you down? Can you tell this part, how it feels ... when you shut me down like that, I feel so ...?*
Clara:	*I don't know how I feel.*
Therapist:	*...So ... you feel nothing ...?*
Clara:	*Yeah I don't feel anything.*
Therapist:	*It does its job well then! I can see that. What does it mean for you? For your life?*
Clara:	*Well, I feel like it helps to feel nothing, like it keeps me safe. But it's weird because I never feel properly safe. I have to always be on guard, keeping an eye out for something that might trigger feelings. I can never relax. It keeps me paralysed.*
Therapist:	*So tell her [indicating coping mode chair], you keep me paralysed. I feel I need you to stay safe, but you also make me feel more unsafe.*
Clara:	*Yes, like you fooled me into thinking you'd protect me, but I feel more scared than ever, like I can't move or think in case feelings come in and I won't be able to cope.*
Therapist:	*Can you tell this part ... what it is that you need from them right now in this moment?*
Clara:	*I don't know; I feel like I can't fight it. [Flipping to express the resignation of a helpless mode.]*
Therapist:	*Yeah ... it's too much. Kind of like: "You win".*
Clara:	*Yeah, but I know that's not really what I want.*
Therapist:	*Ok ... what would it be like to tell that part of you: This is not what I want. I want ...*
Clara [tentatively]:	*A break.*
Therapist:	*Yeah, a break. ... Can you tell that part of you? I need you to give me a break.*
Clara:	*I don't need your help any more.*
Therapist:	*Tell her why.*
Clara [more assertively now]:	*You just make things worse. I see you're trying to help and hear you when you say that you're doing it because you're concerned about what will happen if you don't, but the way things are isn't helping me either. I just need you to let me try.*
Therapist:	*Can you tell her this again ... I need you to stop and let me try to feel.*
Clara:	*Stop it! Back off and let me feel.*
Therapist:	*How do you feel, as you say this? – Back off, let me feel.*
Clara:	*It's scary, but I do really want to explore my feelings more. I feel I need to.*
Therapist:	*So, can you tell her this? I'm scared, but I need to do this.*

Table 7.3 Stages in the Two-chair Work with Coping Modes Task

Stage	Chair	Description	Useful Therapist Prompts
1. **Identify the Marker & Initiate the Task** *Can We Try Something?*	Self chair	Client is caught in a coping mode and exhibiting associated beliefs or behaviours, e.g. Detached Protector blocking feelings.	
2. **Enact the Coping mode** *What Does the Coping Mode Say?*	Coping mode chair	Enact the coping mode. Bring attention to the act (e.g. blocking emotion). Highlight the function (e.g. to protect the self). Amplify the threat of it not being there (e.g. everyone will be there).	"How is it that you block yourself? Can you show me what you do?" "Tell her what will go badly if she doesn't listen to you."
3. **Self Responds to the Coping Mode** *What Does It Feel Like for the Coping Mode to Do This to You?*	Self chair	Elicit initial *emotional* reaction. Notice and name any other coping modes emerging indicative of the client's coping mode patterns, e.g. detached protector triggering a helpless part ("I can't fight it."). Note that clients may report valuing and feeling gratitude to the coping mode – explore the wider impact of the part on the client's life.	"Turn your attention inwards. What happens inside when this happens?" "What is it like for you to be on the receiving end of that?"
4. **Self Expresses Unmet Needs** *What Does the Self Need from he Coping Mode?*	Self chair	Express unmet need. Keep it specific to and directed at the coping mode in the chair not a general need, ideally pertaining to the act of the coping mode (e.g. "I need you to let me have my feelings."). Elaborate the impact on the client's life.	"Can you tell her what you need?"

5. The Coping Mode Responds to the Need *Can the Coping Mode Hear the Need?*	Coping mode chair	If Coping mode **shows compassion & a desire to stop** – this is usually accompanied by fear of what will happen and uncertainty of how to let go.	"How do you respond to this? How do you feel about her as she tells you how you impact her life?"
		If Coping mode shows **no compassion & refusal to stop** – validate the restated function and the associated vulnerability naming the emotions of the Coping mode (e.g. fear).	
Stage 6. Working towards the Healthy Adult and New Boundaries: Negotiation & Integration *Can the Healthy Adult Begin to Be Present?*	Self chair	**Acceptance** (If coping mode showed compassion) – let it in and reflect what it feels like to receive it, explore compromises (e.g. letting emotion in sometimes in safer places).	**Acceptance** – "Can you let that in? What do you think can happen from here? Is there any way to negotiate?" **Assertive Anger** – "What's your response when that part of you rejects what you need without a second thought? How do you feel about that?"
		Assertive Anger (If coping mode shows no compassion) – respond to the non-compassion by stating again the need, often now connecting with assertive anger of the Healthy Adult.	
Debrief	Self chair	(a) Client reflects. (b) Therapist deeply validates any shifts/non-shifts and praises work done. (c) Make links back to the formulation, particularly add any new information revealed about this coping mode to description of parts. (d) Decide on appropriate action (e.g. homework).	

Clara: *I know you are scared, and I am scared too. But it's something we have to do if we are ever going to move forward. I'd like for us to work together. I think we can help each other ... keep the feelings balanced, instead of eliminated.*

Therapist: *Can you tell her what this would look like?*

Clara: *Well, I'm going to let my feelings out a bit in places where it feels more safe ... like tell my therapist what I'm feeling and try to stay with my feelings for longer here.*

Working for Optimal Emotion Regulation

Helpful emotional experience and regulation is a balance; it requires acknowledging and expressing emotions to enable processing, but not becoming so overwhelmed by them that we cannot function. As we have discussed throughout Phase 3, connection with emotion is only possible if therapists can find ways to support clients to overcome avoidance and over-regulation. Some emotion regulation strategies and associated teachings of emotion regulation skills used in therapy can serve to feed in to coping modes and their behaviours, e.g. distraction techniques offering more behavioural fodder for a Detached Protector. This can have a somewhat useful albeit limited function; indeed, not all coping modes are equally unhelpful, and we all use them from time to time. People with anorexia and neurodivergent people can rely heavily on particular emotion regulation strategies with a lack of flexibility and, in particular, those strategies which may be more unhelpful (Cai et al., 2018; Oldershaw et al., 2015). SPEAKS therapists will by now have noticed with their clients that coping modes as emotion regulation strategies ultimately take people away from the core pain and anguish felt by the Little Self and are also not adequate to soothe it. Therefore, they ultimately 'miss the mark' in the short-term and are unhelpful in the long term.

Throughout therapy we develop emotion regulation as a meta-task running through all tasks and seen as the 'master process' (Elliott & Greenberg, 2021), promoting this ability through connection with and transformation of emotion experience. Alongside this, we support regulation, moderation, and containing of a very strong (secondary) emotion, but not the blocking or squashing of it entirely. We also want to respond and offer the pain something soothing and caring, especially when it relates to the core pain of the Little Self. In this section, we explore ways in which we might first *moderate overwhelming emotions* and then how we might *soothe, hold and contain the core pain and anguish of the Little Self.*

Moderating Overwhelming Emotions in the Present

Where clients are currently feeling vulnerable and raw, behavioural strategies to soothe and emotional holding responses from therapists in the moment can be most useful. Before selecting specific techniques to offer to clients, it can be helpful for the therapist to hold in mind what the soothing or regulating task they are considering ultimately achieves and whether it feeds into a coping mode; in other words, they consider whether it is a beneficial tool for their client. It is important that this work does not come across as trying to erase or minimise emotion. Talking about any approaches as strategies that can help clients 'take care of and calm' their emotions can offer a useful frame.

Client's Own Strategies

Therapists should check out a client's self-soothing repertoire early on in therapy, asking how clients typically manage emotion in the initial few sessions. It is important that self-soothing tasks match the needs of the client, and so it is useful to explore a client's naturally occurring self-soothing strategies (listening to music, moderate exercise, artistic pursuits) and to be curious about these and to build on them before introducing new ideas. Links can be made back to coping modes, reflecting on how useful that may make them in the long term and that using them with meta-awareness and choice is most helpful. Once established, these tools can be drawn upon whenever a client becomes dysregulated.

Somatic Resources

Clients who are neurodivergent may engage in specific coping behaviours to self-regulate. Stimming (short for self-stimulatory behaviour) enables sensory and emotion regulation. The stereotypical form of this is 'hand-flapping', but it can involve a range of behaviours, most commonly foot/finger tapping or jiggling, repetitive movements (including rocking), nail biting, and twirling or playing with hair. Stimming provides relief from excessive sensory stimulation, but also from high levels of emotion, including uncertainty and anxiety (Leekam et al., 2011). Autistic adults have highlighted stimming as an important adaptive mechanism to soothe or communicate intense emotions or thoughts (Kapp et al., 2019). In the context of therapy, it affords a useful resource for neurodivergent clients in self-soothing. Therapists should explore, validate and encourage client's stimming behaviours as needed in sessions, including the use of 'fidget toys' or other tools. If therapists see clients using a 'stimming' behaviour they can suggest the increased use of this.

Indeed, these naturally occurring resources arise for all clients (including neurotypical clients) and a therapist can build on or develop with their client a repertoire of somatic resources. Often, especially during work with the Little Self, we might observe our client place a *hand towards their heart* or other small gestures such as stroking their arm to gently regulate. A repetitive stroking of the arm can be encouraged to become bigger and more deliberate, an emerging rocking motion can be experimented with until it feels like the optimal level of soothing movement. A therapist draws attention to these actions and guides the client to deepen and build on these naturally occurring resources ("How does it feel when you place your hand to your heart? Maybe try gently rubbing this area and see how this feels."). Then we can draw on it at other times when they may find it harder to access ("Maybe this is a moment where placing your hand to your heart may help. Little Clara needs to know that you are there for her.").

Other somatic resources, including grounding and orientation, movement, and breath can also be drawn upon, as with other therapeutic approaches.

Soothe, Hold and Contain the Core Pain and Anguish of the Little Self

Once the client has accessed core pain, resources to soothe that anguish whilst increasing safety to maintain the connection to the Little Self supports client's continued processing and builds their emotion self-regulation capability. This can include the use of the therapeutic relationship, soothing imagery and 'audio flash cards' to directly reassure the Little Self and core pain.

Therapeutic Relationship

If client is connected to the core pain of Little Self (as opposed to overwhelming secondary emotion), attempting to respond to the marker of vulnerability with a soothing task could leave the client feeling abandoned or as if their pain is too great for the therapist to handle. One way to facilitate optimal emotion regulation in the moment-to-moment of therapy is for the therapist to employ a gentle emotion coaching stance with empathic attunement (see Chapter 6). Finding words for and an understanding of emotion has, in itself, an emotion regulating effect. Therefore, via the coaching stance, client emotion regulation and soothing abilities are encouraged over time, and as such, clients learn to tolerate and self-regulate emotional pain in an important change process inherent in SPEAKS.

Other ways in which we use the therapeutic relationship is through the use of 'limited reparenting' (Andriopoulou, 2021) to match the attachment unmet need associated with the core pain which has been accessed (See Table 5.1, Chapter 5). In the case of sadness/loneliness-based core pain, unmet needs are for connection and care, and additional contact between sessions can be indicated. It can be in the form of brief emails to let clients know that you are thinking of them and holding them and their Little Self in mind.

Self-soothing Imagery

Self-soothing imagery exercises are particularly useful to support a client's sense of safety and emotional acceptance. The purpose of these tasks is to optimally resource clients so that they feel safe enough and soothed enough to be able to 'stay with' some of the deeper emotional states that may be encountered and worked with during therapy. They can be useful early on in therapy or just whenever the client seems able. A well-known example of this is 'safe place' imagery (imagining and entering a safe place). Here we describe an alternative to this: 'safe bubble'. As a therapist you may have experience of similar exercises that you feel are appropriate for your clients and can bring into your work during SPEAKS.

These tasks can be introduced in session as a form of guided practice with the therapist guiding the client. If experienced as valuable, they can then be audio or video recorded (with the client's consent) to their phone. The client can then be invited to integrate the guided practice into their lives on a regular basis and/or at times when they feel distressed and/or within therapy sessions when they feel triggered. An important part of 'limited reparenting' is scaffolding clients to build their own resources to respond to their own core pain and so the amount of therapist involvement in directing these exercises may lessen over time.

Detailed Instructions for Safe Bubble Exercise

The 'Safe Bubble' exercise meets the need for 'safe boundaries and limits' where these have been transgressed, as well as being useful for clients who cannot picture a safe place. The membrane of the bubble can provide a layer around the Self that is a necessary ingredient for safety where individuals have endured interpersonal trauma. A safe bubble can also be useful in the context of therapy sessions, especially when a two-chair critical voice task reveals an annihilating Self-Critic and that task must be suspended or, as a minimum, some containment introduced.

Generate the Image of the Bubble

Close your eyes or look down and take a few deep slow breaths. Feel your body and mind and notice any sensations you may have.

Now, try to imagine that you are surrounded by a huge transparent bubble. It is a beautiful magic bubble that contains you and can protect you from anything outside of it.

No unhelpful critic voices can get through the walls of the bubble. It is unbreakable – no one can get in, but you can walk in and out of it if you need to or take it with you as you move.

Encourage the Client's Ownership of the Bubble and Enhance Their Sense of Safety

Feel the comfort, safety and warmth of the bubble. Make it your own. It is entirely your space and no one else's; make it is as safe as you can. It's a safe space designed entirely for you and with your needs in mind.

You can make it as big or small as you want, and bring into it any comfort objects that you like, anything you want that will be soothing to you and help you feel stronger and more safe. Nothing that can harm you can be brought into the bubble.

Notice what's inside the bubble. What do you see/hear/smell? Is there anything comforting you can touch now? Would you like to stay alone in the bubble or bring someone in? Is there anything else that you would like to add to make it a perfect special place of yours?

Explore All Senses in the Bubble and Let Feelings of Safety In

How do you feel now, as you sit in this bubble, what do you hear, what do you see? Where is that sense of safety located in your body?

See if you can really build on that sense of safety, really embody all of what the safe bubble provides for you, try to make the sense of warmth and safety as present as you can.

Bring the Safety into Your Present Day

When the client has spent some time in the bubble, encourage them to open their eyes and debrief the exercise.

When it feels right, open your eyes and try to bring the sense of safety into the present day. If you wish, keep the bubble around you. Or you can call up the bubble in your mind's eye to surround you whenever you need it. It is your safe bubble for you to use however suits you best.

Building on Soothing Imagery

As a therapist you can use your creativity to build on these exercises as you think is appropriate. For example, it may be that the safe place exercise can be used to begin self-compassion work. Clara's safe place was her grandma's living room. In her image, her grandma was there with her. Once the therapist had completed the initial exercise, they were able to draw on her internalised grandma's voice. Clara was able to reflect on what would Grandma say to her; what would Grandma want her to know; what does Grandma value in Clara? Later they built on this further using the two-chair self-compassion exercise in Phase 4 (Chapter 8), with Grandma in the chair offering compassion to Clara in the first instance. Slowly they built up to Clara being able to offer herself compassion as her Healthy Adult further emerged. Soothing imagery can also bring a sense of containment to therapy sessions and support client's sense of safety in exploring emotion in the space. At times when she was feeling vulnerable, both Clara and her therapist entered the safe bubble together to give a layer of distance from the harsh critic and enable Clara to more freely explore emotional vulnerability.

Audio Flash Card

Flash Cards have been traditionally a key tool of Cognitive Behavioural Therapy, designed to challenge core beliefs and dysfunctional assumptions underpinning unhelpful behaviours and to begin to orient individuals towards change. In this traditional form, they are usually written out as a paper flash card that the client can keep with them. In SPEAKS, we find that flash cards can also be valuable resources for challenging over-reliance on coping modes and for speaking directly to the Little Self. To increase the relational and emotional heat of this intervention, we suggest audio recording the flash card to the client's phone (with their consent), either in the therapist voice (if there is a reparenting aim, or if the client's Healthy Adult is hard to reach at this point) or with the client's voice (such as later in therapy as they build their own Healthy Adult to guide them). Audio flash cards also function as a transitional object, for example, when the therapist is on a break, or the client has some challenges ahead and values a reminder that they are held in mind. Thus, it might be that during the earlier stages of therapy where the goals are about deepening emotional and relational connection and bypassing coping modes, it is most effective to have the therapist's voice on the recording, and with time, this can be 'handed over' to the client's Healthy Adult.

It is useful to agree the aim of the flash card and to elicit the language that will be used. The audio recording is made together in session and played through to check it feels right to the client and speaks to the mode in the way intended.

Clara's Audio Flash Card

Clara and her therapist developed an audio flash card to support her to come alongside her core pain of her abandoned Little Self when this is triggered by her partner going away, rather than to block this pain via a coping mode. It is important to use the client's language for their experience when they are in the identified mode. In this case, when Clara is in touch with her Little Self and the core pain of lonely abandonment.

> **Right now I feel** ... *sad, frightened, overwhelmed, desolate and like everyone has disappeared and they will never return.*

> **This is because** ... *when I was younger, I had many experiences of those who were meant to be there for me leaving abruptly or not being attuned to my suffering such that feelings became threatening and unmanageable, and I learnt to cut off from these feelings via my Emotion Squasher or Perfectionist Overcontroller.*

Note that here the client orients to historical information that provides a compassionate frame for why these schemata, modes, and feeling states are so intense and why there may be a pull towards a coping mode. Of course, this awareness must have already been reached during therapy and the flash card merely builds on this, extending it beyond the therapy space into the client's life.

> **What I know now is** ... *that there are many people who love me and care about me and want the best for me. Plus, I have parts of me, my Balanced Clara, who can 'hold' me when I feel these feelings and help me respond in soothing and containing ways so that I can hear what I need and respond with patience and*

kindness. Even if I squash my feelings with a coping mode, I know that the hurt remains.

Here the aim is to provide a prompt for a different self-to-self relationship. In this case, Clara is being guided to allow her Healthy Adult in and avoid interrupting her connection with emotion (via a coping mode).

So what I can do now is *… take out photos of my partner and remind myself of his continued existence even when he is not physically here. Then I can try to calm and connect with Little Me, using my hand placed to my heart to send her a message to remind her she is seen and valued and loved. I can remind myself I don't need to squash my emotions right now and can use the safe bubble or cuddles with my dog for a few moments to feel safe with my feelings.*

The aim here is to offer around three concrete behavioural suggestions to fully anchor the Healthy Adult and meet some of the needs of and scaffold the emotional processing of the Little Self.

Additional Considerations, Including for Neurodivergent Clients

For some clients who have endured trauma, the word 'safety' and/or the practice of using imagery to build a safe place or bubble is highly triggering – to be safe would be to let go of the vigilance and watchfulness that helped them survive their earlier lives. This may be particularly true of neurodivergent people. In this case, building safety takes time and typically occurs between two people; the therapeutic relationship may be the first encounter of interpersonal safety. This cannot be bypassed, and it requires a slower pace and patience. It may be that the above tasks are not fitting for these clients. For other clients there is a sense of the partialness of these tasks or sometimes anger at building safety 'artificially'. These are real and understandable reactions, and it is important to validate the anger, regret, and disappointment that safety was not present at a time when they most needed it.

Moving from Phase 3 (Deepening to Core Pain) to Phase 4 (Resolving Core Pain)

Phase 3 moves into Phase 4 when core pain has been experienced and elaborated. Of note is that Phase 3 flows into Phase 4 seamlessly in a process of emotion transformation with some tasks (e.g. chair work with the broader Critic; float back) straddling both phases. Furthermore, there will be considerable movement back and forth between these phases.

Once this core pain has begun to be uncovered and – via the therapeutic relationship and self-soothing work – there has been an established sense of safety in working with core pain and unmet need, you are moving into Phase 4: Resolving Core Pain.

References

Andriopoulou, P. (2021). Healing attachment trauma in adult psychotherapy: The role of limited reparenting. *European Journal of Psychotherapy & Counselling, 23*(4), 468–482.

Cai, R. Y., Richdale, A. L., Uljarević, M., Dissanayake, C., & Samson, A. C. (2018). Emotion regulation in autism spectrum disorder: Where we are and where we need to go. *Autism Research, 11*(7), 962–978.

Elliott, R., & Greenberg, L. (2021). *Emotion-focused counselling in action.* Sage.

Elliott, R., Watson, J. C., Goldman, R. N., & Greenberg, L. S. (2004). *Learning emotion-focused therapy: The process-experiential approach to change.* American Psychological Association.

Greenberg, L. S. (2021). *Changing emotion with emotion: A practitioner's guide.* American Psychological Association.

Greenberg, L. S., & Elliott, R. (2012). Corrective experience from a humanistic–experiential perspective. In L. G. Castonguay & C. E. Hill (Eds.), *Transformation in psychotherapy: Corrective experiences across cognitive behavioral, humanistic, and psychodynamic approaches* (pp. 85–101). American Psychological Association. https://doi.org/10.1037/ 13747-006.

Heath, G., & Startup, H. (2020). Creative methods with coping modes and chair work. In G. Heath & H. Startup (Eds.). *Creative Methods in Schema Therapy* (pp. 178–194). Routledge.

Holmes, E. A., Arntz, A., & Smucker, M. R. (2007). Imagery rescripting in cognitive behaviour therapy: Images, treatment techniques and outcomes. *Journal of Behavior Therapy and Experimental Psychiatry, 38*(4), 297–305.

Kapp, S. K., Steward, R., Crane, L., Elliott, D., Elphick, C., Pellicano, E., & Russell, G. (2019). "People should be allowed to do what they like": Autistic adults' views and experiences of stimming. *Autism, 23*(7), 1782–1792.

Leekam, S. R., Prior, M. R., & Uljarevic, M. (2011). Restricted and repetitive behaviors in autism spectrum disorders: a review of research in the last decade. *Psychological Bulletin, 137*(4), 562–593.

Loomes, R., & Bryant-Waugh, R. (2021). Widening the reach of family-based interventions for Anorexia Nervosa: autism-adaptations for children and adolescents. *Journal of Eating Disorders, 9*, 1–11.

Malik-Smith, S., Papastavrou Brooks., C., Callanan, M., Pascual-Leone, A. & Oldershaw, A. (in prep) The process of emotion change associated with recovery from anorexia nervosa.

Oldershaw, A., Lavender, T., Sallis, H., Stahl, D., & Schmidt, U. (2015). Emotion generation and regulation in anorexia nervosa: A systematic review and meta-analysis of self-report data. *Clinical Psychology Review, 39*, 83–95.

Simpson, S., & Arntz, A. (2020). Core principles of imagery. In G. Heath & H. Startup (Eds.), *Creative Methods in Schema Therapy* (pp. 93–107). Routledge.

Timulak, L., & Keogh, D. (2020). Emotion-focused therapy: A transdiagnostic formulation. *Journal of Contemporary Psychotherapy, 50*(1), 1–13.

Chapter 8

Phase 4

Resolving Core Pain

Once individuals begin to connect with and express core pain associated with their Little Self then Phase 4 of Specialist Psychotherapy with Emotion for Anorexia in Kent and Sussex (SPEAKS) can be progressed. Phase 4 seeks to engage clients to resolve core pain in a process of *emotion transformation: changing emotion with emotion*. This change process gives rise to a new experiences leading to an integrated and transformed state with new perspectives on the self and others. Self-compassion can be best developed during this phase, harnessed using tasks for *building self-compassion*. As new meanings and self-narratives emerge, they strengthen the Healthy Adult and facilitate a reintegration of self that is more needs led, emotionally connected and resilient (the 'Real Me').

Emotion Transformation: Changing Emotion with Emotion

Common to Schema Therapy (ST), Emotion Focused Therapy (EFT), and SPEAKS, core pain is understood to have emerged within a context of early life (often chronic) unmet need. Core pain experienced later in life reflects a 'flood of activation' including the triggering of these 'emotional memories' and associated schema, as well as linked behavioural and bodily responses, such that the emotional states become chronically felt (Flanagan et al., 2020) and become easily triggered 'story of my life' feelings (Elliott et al., 2004). As highlighted throughout this guidebook, other parts of the self emerge in life to attempt to express distress associated with unmet needs or manage the associated core pain (such as coping modes), and these can be over-relied upon in adult life.

For people with anorexia nervosa (AN) and other eating disorders (EDs), the Eating Disorder Part (EDP) may first present itself as a best attempt to meet these needs, but over time, these limited ways of being fail to hit the mark and only serve to maintain the core pain. By moving beyond the global distress of secondary emotions (e.g. guilt) or secondary processes (e.g. anxiety around eating and body image), clients access, differentiate, and express core pain (e.g. shame

DOI: 10.4324/9781003468349-10

and lonely abandonment) and identify and express associated needs (e.g. *"I want to be accepted, seen/heard and loved just as I am."*) (SPEAKS Phases 1–3). This expression leads to a perspective shift in relation to the unmet needs and vulnerability linked to primary adaptive emotions such as assertive anger (e.g. *"I deserved to be loved and accepted."*), grief/hurt (e.g. *"I miss and grieve that Little Me didn't have that acceptance and loving experience."*), and/or soothing and compassion (e.g. *"I can feel loved and accepted now."*) giving rise to the transformed state of agency and efficacy; an integrated 'Real Me'. This emotion transformation process has been observed within session and across therapy for a range of clinical presentations (Greenberg & Pascual-Leone, 2024; Keogh & Timulak, 2023; Pascual-Leone, 2018) and is the process we seek to facilitate in Phase 4 of SPEAKS therapy.

Phase 4 involves the 'Float Back with Rescripting' task (Simpson and Arntz, 2020) affording clients an opportunity to further connect with the core pain of the Little Self in episodic memories and identify unmet needs, facilitating a 'corrective emotional experience'. The 'Unfinished Business' task enables expression of core pain and unmet need in the context of internalised (developmental) relationships in which it developed, leading to emergence of the Healthy Adult and shifts in views of the Self or Other. When the 'Float Back with Rescripting' task is revisited, the Healthy Adult entering the memory can offer compassion to the Little Self but also further connect with primary adaptive emotions in the face of the remembered unmet need and use those emotions to guide action tendencies in meeting need.

Task: Float Back with Rescripting

The 'Float Back with Rescripting' task aims to change the emotional tone of a painful memory through the meeting of client needs. This affords an opportunity to transform their emotional experience. It is most appropriate with earlier developmental memories and can be used to provide alternative emotional 'memories' that a client can access, to counter existing damaging and painful memories of childhood experiences (Simpson and Arntz, 2020). As described in the initial 'Float Back' task in Phase 3 (Chapter 7), this task involves connecting with a present day painful familiar feeling (primary maladaptive emotion: core pain) as an 'affect bridge' to 'float back' to an earlier memory with the same or similar feeling attached. Where this task differs is in the rescripting element. In short, 'Float Back with Rescripting' involves first elaborating and then 'entering' an early memory and altering events such that the unmet needs of the child within it can be met to some degree and importantly, the rescript comes to a close when these needs are met sufficiently and the individual feels safe.

Whilst this may appear to have some overlap with Cognitive Behavioural Therapy (CBT) rescripting (such as that used in Trauma Focused CBT), there are differences. Here, the therapist may have a key role in the reparative function of the rescripted memory, drawing on their 'reparenting' stance. The worked-on image or memory also need not be intrusive in the client's mind but can rather be associated with painful emotions attached to unmet needs. The therapist entering a memory rescript can nurture, comfort, and care for a child, directly confront an abuser, protect the child from harm, and remove him/her to safety. Here is a process of reattribution, emotional processing, and meeting of the need (e.g. receiving care) (Arntz, 2012; Simpson & Arntz, 2020); this gives rise to an emerging experience of primary adaptive emotion (e.g. soothing and love) changing the emotional but also the cognitive meaning (e.g. "I deserved care, and I can feel care.") at the level of the Little Self. These feelings and reattributions can be further generalised in subsequent work, contributing to the emergence of the Healthy Adult and a transformed sense of self. The use of this task in conjunction with the 'Unfinished Business' task engages both verbal and visual processing of core pain, which may afford more powerful change opportunities and supports a breadth of processing styles.

Detailed Guidelines for Float Back with Rescripting Task

The initial five steps are the same as the original 'Float Back' task, with the addition of 'Rescripting' later in the task (See Table 8.1 and Float Back task in Phase 3 for details of additional considerations in applying the task).

Table 8.1 Stages in the Float Back with Rescripting Task

Stage	Description	Key Therapist Responses
Stage 1. Identify the Marker & Initiate the Task – *Can We Try Something?*	Client recalls memories of relationships which feel traumatic due to core pain attached or a specific incident which has happened recently where core pain was triggered.	
Stage 2. Elaborate Details of the Memory – *Tell Me More about When This Feeling Came*	• Describe the memory in detail.	• Try to recall a recent time when you felt in touch with that same feeling and walk me through it.
Stage 3. Connect with and Deepen the Core Pain – *Can We Make This Feeling 'Bigger'?*	• Focus inwards. • Support the 'felt sense' of the emotion. • Make the feeling 'big' to deepen connection.	• Tell me where in your body these feelings are located. • How would you describe the way you feel right now?

Table 8.1 (Continued)

Stage	Description	Key Therapist Responses
Stage 4. Float Back – *Is There an Earlier Memory That Fits with This Feeling?*	• Hold on to the feeling and clear mind of current memory. • Find an earlier memory with this same feeling.	• Stay with these feelings but erase the present memory from your mind. • Try to find an earlier memory or state with these same feelings attached.

Stage 5. Elaborate the Memory or Association – *Tell Me More about the Earlier Memory of this Feeling*	• Get a detailed description of the new memory accessed.
	• Get a description of the client, including age in the memory, and who else was present.
		• Please can you describe the scene to me?
		  Who is there?
		  What is happening?
		  What is the worst bit of it/most painful part?
		  What did you need in the image?

Stage 6. Enter the Image for Rescripting – *What Is the Need and How Can It Be Met?*	• With client permission, therapist enters the image. • Therapist recognises and validates core pain. • Therapist goes some way to meet the original unmet need in imagery. • Revisiting this task later, client's own Healthy Adult may enter the scene.	• What do you need to feel better/safe in this situation?
Debrief	(a) Client reflects. (b) Therapist deeply validates any shifts/non-shifts and praises work done. (c) Make links back to the formulation. (d) Decide on appropriate action (e.g. homework.)	

Stage 1. Identifying the Marker and Initiating the Task – *Can We Try Something?*

The marker for this task is that a client connects with a core pain that is familiar and a 'bad, stuck' feeling in their life in a recent memory or recalls memories which feel traumatic due to core pain attached.

Stage 2. Evoke and Elaborate the Memory – *Tell Me More about When This Feeling Came*

First the goal is to elaborate the memory attached to this feeling, either the recent one or a past memory in the first person, ideally with eyes closed ("Can you talk me through that experience? Tell me what happened?").

Stage 3. Connect with and Deepen the Core Pain – *Can We Make This Feeling Bigger?*

As the client reaches the point of emotion activation in their description (the 'hot' moment, i.e. when core pain such as shame or lonely abandonment was at its strongest), the client makes this feeling as present and embodied as possible.

Stage 4. Float Back – *Is There an Earlier Memory That Fits with This Feeling?*

Next the client is supported to form an 'affect bridge', using the emotion to 'float back' to access other memories which resonate with these feelings. The goal is to go back as far as possible, giving time and space to drift back with these feelings.

Stage 5. Elaborate the Memory or Association – *Tell Me More about the Memory*

Once a client is ready, and has fallen upon an associated memory or image, they spend time elaborating the scene and who else was there, so that both therapist and client fully and dynamically appreciate it, especially in relation to the unmet needs.

Stage 6. Enter the Image for Rescripting – *What Is the Need and How Can It Be Met?*

Once the image has been activated, the therapist considers whether it might be helpful for them to enter the image and support rescripting. This should be gently and collaboratively discussed with the client. A therapist is guided by the client and simply follows their instructions, doing whatever is necessary in imagery for the needs of the client to be met and for them to feel safe and secure. The therapist adopts a reparenting stance, attuning to the unmet need to nurture, comfort, and care for a child, directly confront an abuser, protect the child from harm, and/or remove him/her to safety. The imagery comes to a close when the client feels safe and secure and the past unmet needs are met.

Debrief

Invite the client to open their eyes and re-orient them to the room. Debrief by asking the client to reflect on how the task felt for them.

(a) **Client reflects.** Client tells therapist what they notice from the task trying to tease out any meaning made. What do they take away? Ask the client to put into a first person 'I' statement (e.g. "I don't deserve to be spoken to like that, I have done nothing wrong; I feel stronger.").

(b) **Therapist deeply validates any shifts/non-shifts, praises work done and prizes emotion shared.**

(c) **Make links back to the formulation.** Clearly connect what has emerged to the mode map and highlight where the new experiences indicate change has occurred.

(d) **Decide on any appropriate action, ideas of different experiences or actions that might be tried between sessions.** Try to keep this collaborative and client directed. Examples include learning to identify and express needs to others (via an emotion and needs diary and behavioural experiments).

Clara

Clara worked on a recent memory of arranging a social gathering with some colleagues from work. She had sent out a message via text for a gathering at a local pub and had booked a table and gone along early to be there as host and to meet with whoever came. Despite lots of confirmations of attendance, on the night only one person showed up, leaving Clara feeling crushed, embarrassed, and with a sense of over-responsibility for the experience of that one person. She vividly recalled this event with her therapist and the sense of crushing shame as she realised others were not coming. In imagery, her therapist used the sense of her quite visceral shame/embarrassment/burden and guided Clara to 'stay with' these feelings, embody them, and make them bold, to really take in this felt sense. She was then guided to 'let go' of the current memory but 'hold on' to the painful feelings of shame/embarrassment/burden and 'float back' to a time earlier in her life when she may have felt something similar.

Clara initially said she had a couple of associated memories, so her therapist guided her to elaborate the earliest. Clara recounted a scene at school when she was seven years old. She had attended an after-school club but was left in a room all by herself, just waiting endlessly, because her mother had forgotten to pick her up. She remembered it getting dark outside and the sense of shame/embarrassment but also a crushing aloneness in the awareness that everyone else had been picked up, and now she was the only one alone and waiting. She felt deep shame that she was holding up the teachers who wanted to get home themselves and a sense of responsibility. Her therapist gently suggested that no little child should be alone and sad carrying the burden of adult mistakes (her mother's mistake) and asked whether she might enter the image.

Her therapist asked Little Clara in the image 'what she needed' to feel better in this situation. Clara replied that she wanted to be distracted and not just left waiting by herself; she then wanted to be taken home and cared for and looked after. Her therapist responded in imagery in an attuned and needs-led manner by entering the image and being guided by Clara to sit alongside her, following which, the therapist suggested they play a game together of her choosing. The image of them playing gymnastics outside in the open air was elaborated and deepened such that shared joy between them was present. The therapist in the image then said she could get the bus with Clara to get her safely home. The therapist checked in continually with the needs of Little Clara who said that she felt safer, calmer, and engrossed in the joy of the interest the therapist showed in her and in the games they were playing together. She no longer felt embarrassed or a burden but seen and appreciated.

The therapist checked in with Clara about any residual worries she had. Clara said that she worried her mother would never return. Her therapist responded to this core terror linked to abandonment and they agreed to end the image with the two of them reuniting with her mother at home. The therapist stayed with Clara until she felt safe and cared for and reassured that her mother understood the impact her forgetting had had on Little Clara. Clara was guided to deepen the feelings of joy, safety, and containment throughout her body, and the exercise ended with Clara being guided to open her eyes, return to the present moment, and bring with her those feelings of connected contentment.

During the debrief Clara could link the pain of not being held in mind by her busy and preoccupied mother with the sense of shame, loneliness, and burden she often experienced when she felt 'not seen' or abandoned by others. She was also aware of her habitual pattern of blocking this pain via her overcompensator and avoidant coping modes, in particular her EDP. Here Clara was able to connect with her Healthy Adult part, Balanced Clara. She and her therapist made an audio flash card voice note at the end of the session to Little Clara from her own Healthy Adult, reminding her that she is loved and cared for and her needs are safely held in mind.

Task: Unfinished Business

The 'Empty Chair for Unfinished Business' task was originally developed from Gestalt principles (Perls et al., 1966) to resolve and to move on from past hurt and grief in interpersonal relationships. Building on this work, the field of EFT has updated and shaped the 'Unfinished Business' task utilising change process research to delineate the steps to resolution (Greenberg & Malcolm, 2002).

The 'Unfinished Business' task is used when the client expresses a lingering unresolved negative feeling towards an important or significant Other. It can relate to both past and present unresolved relational issues. Whilst often relating to developmental relationships, recent and current relationships with important others (such as partners, children) can influence client vulnerabilities or exacerbate historical core pain. These painful interpersonal experiences further shape coping and critic modes and trigger core pain. It may be that the task is first used in response to a marker about a current relational issue or a past relationship that is meaningful but not the most significant in the client's life (e.g. a teacher as opposed to a parent). The task involves placing an imagined and internalised sense of the significant Other in an empty chair and engaging in 'conversation' to identify, elaborate, and express previously disowned feelings and needs. Greenberg & Malcolm (2002) found that expressing previously unmet interpersonal needs, shifting the view of the Other whilst affirming themselves, alongside either understanding or holding the Other accountable were fundamental to resolving these stuck patterns.

In SPEAKS we conceptualise this as an emergence of the Healthy Adult, who can offer adaptive emotions of self-compassion and also use assertive anger to set clear and helpful boundaries.

Detailed Guidelines for Unfinished Business (Empty Chair) Task

Below are detailed notes on the 'Unfinished Business' task and what may emerge or be required from the therapist in each step (adapted from Elliott & Greenberg, 2021; Elliott et al., 2004; Timulak & Keogh, 2022; summarised in Table 8.3).

Stage 1. Identify the Marker and Initiate the Task – Can We Try Something?

The marker for this task is a lingering unresolved negative feeling towards an important or significant Other. In simple terms, it is commonly observed as the client expressing blame, complaint, or hurt about somebody specific.

It is likely that prior to this task a client will already have linked core pain to experiences with others (especially via 'Float Back' tasks) and therefore will have explored previous relationships in which this familiar feeling has been evoked. As such it might have been agreed in a previous session that you will further explore particular relationship(s) here.

Stage 2. Express Initial Feelings towards the Other – Tell Them How You Feel.

SENSE THE OTHER

The task requires the client to turn their chair to face another empty chair and imagine or evoke a sense of the person they have unresolved feelings towards sitting in front of them. Ideally, they do not spend too long elaborating or picturing the Other, which can take the client into their head; however, some clients do find it hard to imagine and make contact and need support to deepen this process, such as what the Other might be wearing, the way they are sitting, how old they are (is it the current them or a past them?), their facial expression, or even using pictures or objects as representation if needed.

EXPRESS CURRENT FEELINGS

As soon as the client seems to have a felt sense of the Other, the therapist guides them to their internal experience and immediate feelings.

- "Let's try something. … Can you imagine your mum sitting in that chair opposite you? Just picture her there."

- "What happens inside when you see her there?"
- "Can you tell her, when I see you there I feel ...?"

The therapist as emotion coach guides the client to 'look inside', exploring, naming, and expressing aspects of their internal emotional experience (see Chapter 5. Phase 1).

EXPRESS UNRESOLVED FEELINGS (BE SPECIFIC)

Gradually the client is supported in the unfolding of painful emotion and associated experiences to enable elaboration and expression of feelings about the perceived past injury and/or painful experience of the Other. The client can be helped to use the words that they used when first telling you about it. Evoking a specific incident or memory and being specific can be helpful – "I felt so ... when you ..."

> Clara: You were always too busy when I wanted to talk about the bullying. And it was like you thought I was overreacting or being too sensitive. You were always so busy and often forgot about or failed to see what I was going through. You just weren't interested in me and how I felt.

Stage 3. Enact the Other – *How Does the Attachment Other Respond to Feelings?*

BE THE OTHER

The client switches chairs and enacts the harsh, hurtful, or complacent Other. The goal here is to elicit more clearly the behaviours that were hurtful or difficult for the client. This in turn further evokes the client's responding emotions. They may need encouragement from the therapist to be specific and not talk in generalised terms.

LOOK FOR IMPLICIT MEANING AND EMOTION

Therapists should look for the *implicit meaning* in the message given and encourage its expression ("What was the message given?"). Therapists should also look for the *implicit* (Other's) *emotion* in the message given and encourage its expression. For example, annoyance, contempt, disinterest, disdain, disgust.

- "It's not just that I don't have enough time for you; it's that you're too needy and too much."
- "My work is more important than you, and you don't deserve my attention, time ... or love ...."

Note this stage is optional, and alternatively, Stage 2 can move straight through to Stage 4. The benefit of this stage is that enacting the Other can support evocation of emotion and connection to Little Self.

Stage 4. React to the Other and Deepen to Little Self and Core Pain – *Can You Tell Him/Her What Hurts the Most?*

When the client has enacted the perceived behaviour and implicit meanings and emotions from the Other, the therapist briefly summarises and asks the client to return to the Self chair. Sometimes therapists can find it hard to judge when to ask the client to move chairs and it can be helpful to hold goals in mind. Being in the 'Other' chair evokes and enhances a client's emotional reactions. Therefore, signs indicating that it can be useful to change back to the Self chair are:

- The Other's message has been specified and amplified.
- The Other is still high in emotional energy, as it is at this point that the emotions of the Little Self are most likely to be evoked.
- The client starts spontaneously speaking as, emotionally responding as, or reflecting the body language of the Little Self.

INITIAL EMOTIONAL REACTION TO THE OTHER

The therapist explores and encourage expressions of pain likely to now connect to a deeper emotional reaction since the core message from the Other has been uncovered. The goal here is to deepen past secondary emotion to the primary core pain of the Little Self.

- "Let those words come over and really hit you …"
- "Can you tell them? When you talk to me like that I feel …"

DEEPEN AND DIFFERENTIATE EMOTION TO ACCESS CORE PAIN OF LITTLE SELF

As in all tasks, when the client is in the Self chair, the therapist's guiding of process is oriented by the emotion response type (secondary, core pain, primary adaptive) and by the part of self who responds.

- "Can you tell her what happens inside you as you hear these words again now?"
- "Can you tell her what it did to you and to how you felt about yourself?"
- "What hurt the most about this?"

The therapist remains empathically attuned, guiding the process of client in dialogue with the Other, utilising a stance of questioning curiosity and reflecting with conjecture, as opposed to stating with knowing, facilitates the gradual uncovering and connecting with emotion. Furthermore, gently affirming emotions can be useful ("It's ok to feel angry.", "Of course you feel angry."). Keeping the client in their current felt sense of emotion without asking too many questions to help them stay in the present tense using 'how' and 'what' questions over 'why' questions and with current experiencing ("How do you feel now, as you are saying this?") and bringing emphasis to poignant feelings ("Say that again, it made me feel …") or making them more vivid ("Be the Little Clara who felt so dismissed and lonely when your Mum wasn't there for you"). It may take several chair swops from stages 3 to 4 to deepen to core pain.

Stage 5. Express the NEED – *Can You Tell Him/Her What the Little You Needed?*

EXPRESS INITIAL NEED

Once the client has deepened to the core pain of Little Self (such as shame or lonely abandonment), the therapist asks the client to express the associated unmet need directly to the Other ("When your mum wasn't there to listen to you, Clara, and you were left feeling so abandoned, what is it that you needed from her? Can you tell her?").

DEEPEN AND ELABORATE THE NEEDS OF THE LITTLE SELF

Clients will often present to the Other with either more anger or more sadness in the first instance, and a therapist supports them to move in a dance between and continually deepening and differentiating the emotions of anger and sadness, "What are you mad about and what are you sad about?", interspersed with "What do you need?" This brings clarity and is key to the emotion transformation process. It can be supported by guiding clients towards what is implicit in what they are saying, particularly where it evokes episodic memories.

- For the client who is expressing sadness/grief: "Tell them everything you missed …"; Then, "What do you need?"
- For the client who is expressing anger: "Tell them everything you resent …"; Then, "What do you need?"

It is important that the need is expressed within the context of the activation of the Little Self with associated vulnerability of core pain stimulated and present, i.e. that it is a 'heartfelt need' (Timulak, 2015). Often when asked to express needs outside of sufficiently activated emotion, clients will respond, "I don't know what I need." Heartfelt needs usually reflect a longing for safety, connection (attachment needs), or acceptance/understanding (identity needs). These needs going chronically unmet are what resulted in development of core pain; therefore, the need naturally follows from the pain.

Therapist: So, I needed you to make space for me to … listen to me? To hear me?

Clara: *I needed you to hear me, for there to be space for me. I felt so lonely and unseen.*

Therapist: *Can you tell her what you missed in not having this need met? Like ...*
                I missed feeling ... feeling known ...?
Clara: *I missed feeling known and understood and wanted.*
Therapist: *Right, and that loss left you feeling so ...?*
Clara: *I felt so lonely and like I didn't matter ... just worthless.*
Therapist   *Say more about what you missed ...?*
Clara: *I missed your time ... I missed knowing I was important to you ... feel-
                ing important and special in your eyes ...I so wanted that [expressing
                sadness]. To have time just the two of us to play together or go shop-
                ping ... to do the things that I wanted ...*
Therapist: *Yes, you were just a little girl and wanted time with your mum that was
                about you.*
Clara: *Yes it was never about me. I should have had that ... I needed that ...*
Therapist: *I deserved that ... I deserved to be special and made time for. ...I
                deserved for it to be about me sometimes. Does this fit? I deserved ...?*
Clara: *I did deserve it. Yes! [moving to some assertive anger] I was so small;
                I deserved my mum and to feel special and loved.*

Stage 6. The Other Responds to the NEED – *Can the Need Be Heard?*

Once the client has connected with the Little Self, activated core pain and expressed associated unmet needs, they return to the Other chair and respond ("What do you feel towards Little Clara, who desperately wants you to see her and love her, just as she is?"). This response is likely to reflect either rejection of the pain/needs or compassion towards the pain/need. As therapist, we are being explorative and there is no 'right' response, but you are probing to see if there is any scope for compassion, for the pain and unmet need to be seen, thereby going some way to meet the need.

Again, this stage is optional, and Stage 5 can move straight through to Stage 7. The benefit of this stage is that enacting the Other here can deepen and consolidate emerging primary emotions.

THE OTHER MAY *SHOW COMPASSION* TO NEEDS

The clear expression of any compassion is encouraged and elaborated, including feelings towards the Little Self.

THE OTHER MAY *SHOW NO COMPASSION* AND REJECT NEEDS

The clear expression and exploration of any rejection is encouraged, followed by an enquiry around what blocks compassion and/or the function of rejection.

- "Tell her: You were always oversensitive and reading too much into everything. I am still not willing to listen to you."

- "What's the message you are giving her when you don't hear her pain and see her needs?" Note that this message may relate to expression of the Other's own vulnerability such as Clara's mum: "I was so overwhelmed with work and struggling to cope, there was just no space for me to take on anything else; I was barely holding myself together." Acknowledging this can diminish the power of the message and decentre it from the client's own sense of defect or inadequacy. For Clara, this led to some assertive anger that her needs (now known and felt to be deserved) were unmet, alongside newly emerging genuine compassion for her struggling mum. Her therapist supported the expression of this in Stage 7.

Stage 7. Emergence of the Healthy Adult – *Do You Connect with Healthy Adult Feelings and Action?*

Stating the unmet need, and feeling sufficiently deserving or entitled to that need, leads to a shift into adaptive emotions of self-compassion, assertive anger, and/or grief for the loss. These emotions enable the continued emergence, validation, and integration of the Healthy Adult who can listen to and take care of the Little Self and vulnerable feelings, hearing and meeting needs. This further adds to a sense of empowerment and supports a sense of wholeness – the 'Real Me'.

ADAPTIVE COMPASSION (IF OTHER *SHOWS COMPASSION*)

When the client moves back to the Self chair, we want them to move to the Healthy Adult to hold, truly experience, and savour any compassion and sense of love and care, exploring associated experiential, emotional, and cognitive shifts, and encourage expression of those (this can be further consolidated by moving at this point to 'Chair Work for Self-compassion' between the Healthy Adult and Little Self; see later in this chapter).

- "Can you let that in?"
- "What happens inside when you hear that response – 'I'm sorry and I love you?' Can you tell her what it's like?"

The witnessing of this by the therapist validates and enhances the experience of being cared for and connected with others (meeting unmet attachment needs). Accessing adaptive emotion, followed by an experience of reconnection and soothing, afford a client an empowerment which is the antidote to the shame of perceived personal inadequacy or the loneliness of feeling unable to be soothed (Greenberg, 2010). In this healing and empowerment, we see the Healthy Adult develop.

ADAPTIVE ANGER (IF OTHER *SHOWS NO COMPASSION*)

If the client as Other shows no compassion and rejects the core pain and needs of the Little Self, the client back in their own chair can further access and express assertive anger in response; they deserved more. Note that here we are encouraging the client to move to the Healthy Adult rather than further access the pain of the Little Self. As such the therapist does not ask the client to look inside at how it feels to have received this response, but rather respond to the non-compassion.

- "What do you say to her when she tells you you're too sensitive and overreacting?"
- "Will you just accept her telling you this and being so dismissive of Little Clara?"

The client can be encouraged to respond as the Healthy Adult.

- "Now I'm an adult, I can see that you were lacking in your role as parent."

The process sought here is one of holding the Other accountable whilst also affirming the Self and the validity of needs and emotions. Clients may not (at first) access the assertive anger of the Healthy Adult and instead express the sadness and grief of the Little Self who has not had their needs heard. They continue to hold on tightly to the longing for this need to be met. The therapist can support the expression of this longing to the Other.

- "I just can't let go of the hope that you'll change/things will be different."
- "I am still longing for you to be the mum I wanted, and I can't let go of that."

This expression can lead to another round of the task moving back to Stage 3 or revisiting in later sessions following more imagery work in 'Float Back'.

ADAPTIVE GRIEF AND LETTING GO

The clear and strong expression of primary adaptive emotions and supporting the emergence of the Healthy Adult who can hold boundaries and offer themself compassion, leads to a new view of the Self and Other. Ultimately this enables the letting go of previously unresolved feelings and needs (or at least reducing the attachment to and pain associated with them) which is where this task resolves. It can take several sessions to achieve this, and as discussed below, this process can be further facilitated by using this task in combination with the 'Float Back with Rescripting' task.

A changed view of the self in the newly felt Healthy Adult can be embedded via gentle exploration and focusing on the felt sense (see also 'Phase 5: The Real Me'). The client moves from fragility to strength, self-efficacy, and empowerment (Sharbanee et al., 2019). Integrating the felt sense and language for this shift are an important aspect of the task.

There can also be a change in the view of the Other, as with Clara who saw her mum's vulnerability. The Other may now be seen as more loving and caring than before or shifted from powerful to weak or from somebody who intended to hurt to somebody who never meant to. The client may be able to access a greater range of memories of the Other, broadening their sense of them and the range of messages they received (good as well as hurtful).

We often see assertive anger or receiving of compassion to be quickly followed by grief at what was deserved but missed, leading to a process of grieving and 'letting go'. Indeed, the letting go of unmet need usually means the loss of something extremely important to the client; it is the letting go of the hope that your needs will be met and letting go of trying to change the past. Therefore, a process of grieving can be crucial. This grieving can be understood as an adaptive sadness, reflecting the lost connection, and can be responded to by allowing its elaboration and expression, whilst offering validation, empathy, and 'limited reparenting'.

Debrief

Once the task is finished, reflecting on the resolution or where the task has reached before the session ends is an important part of the process.

(a) **Client reflects.** Client tells therapist what they notice from the task trying to tease out any meaning made. What do they take away? Ask the client to put into a first person 'I' statement (e.g. "I deserved more."; "I feel sadness."; "I feel empowered.").
(b) **Therapist deeply validates any shifts/non-shifts, praises work done and prizes emotion shared.**
(c) **Make links back to the formulation.**
(d) **Decide on any appropriate action, ideas of different experiences or actions that might be tried between sessions**. Try to keep this collaborative and client directed. Homework that incorporates greater awareness is valuable. This could include making time each day to see if they can connect in an embodied way with the empowered feelings of the Healthy Adult. The client might find it useful to listen out for the feelings they experienced as the Healthy Adult, naming them and tracking in a diary. They might notice what facilitates the connection with these feelings or what gets in the way. For clients who were able to bring self-compassion during the task, they might consider, "What are the ways in which I can try to show myself compassion this week? What would that look like?"

Clara set about writing a letter (unsent) to her mother from her Little Self expressing further the pain associated with the continual abandonments of not being held in mind. She was able to express what she had needed from her, along with putting voice to the disappointment, anger, and grief that resulted from the reality that these needs were not met when she most needed them to be (in childhood). She made a promise to her Little Self to not repeat this pain in the present. This written elaboration supported her processing of new emerging meanings.

Additional Considerations, Including for Neurodivergent Clients

Difficulty Saying Anything Perceived as 'Negative' to an Attachment Figure or in Enacting the Other

When clients are often strongly compliant, it can feel hard to criticise others. It may be that the client speaks in a very matter of fact manner about the other and events that occurred without expressing any associated emotion, suggesting a coping mode is at play such as a strong compliant mode ("It would be wrong to say anything 'bad' about my mum.") or the emotional avoidance of Detached Protector ("I don't feel anything; it's just how it was."). There may be self-interruptions when enacting the other, particularly when, as a therapist, you are encouraging them to explicitly use the tone or the strong words that may only have been implicit. This can feel a shameful process for the client; both in terms of the message about themselves that they are revealing, but also because they may believe it feels critical to express anything about the enacted other that can be negatively perceived. Autistic people with anorexia in particular can be overly empathic to needs and emotions of others (Nimbley et al., 2023). This can be gently named with the client. Any hesitation and uncertainty should be held and validated and the client encouraged to give the task a go with the support of the therapist. It can be helpful to let clients know (where relevant) that it is recognised that the Other was just trying their best, but that does not mean their behaviour did not impact the client, and their feelings matter and should be honoured too.

Clients can also worry that they don't know exactly what the other person would say and this can disproportionately affect neurodivergent people who think concretely and may worry about portraying events accurately. Taking another person's perspective or feeling empathy for their position can be especially difficult if the client is neurodivergent and the other person is neurotypical, or vice versa, as their perceptions and thinking styles differ from one another, reflecting the 'Double Empathy problem' (Milton et al., 2022). Guidance and reassurance is offered that the goal is not to find accuracy in literally how the other might think/respond or in specifically what would/did happen, but in the client's internalisations. Emphasising that we are not seeking to discern and apportion blame or to gain an accurate historical record of events can be particularly important for autistic clients who are more likely to initially interpret the steps of the task literally or with too much focus on details not necessary for task completion, rather than an appreciation of the wider goal of their felt experience. If it is too difficult and impeding the task, embodying the 'other' can be removed from the task.

Difficulty Responding to the Other

It can also be extremely daunting, even terrifying, once the Other has been more firmly activated in the client's mind for the client to respond and they may understandably be hesitant or nervous. When clients are finding it hard to express their needs to the Other, an alternative approach, suggested by Timulak and Keogh (2022), is to ask the client to nominate a different imagined Other who would have had potential to hear their need ("Who would have heard what you would need? Can you tell her what you need when you feel this pain?"). Clients may also be able to tell the therapist what they needed in the first instance. Once the client has experienced expression of the need in this emotionally safer context, they may feel more able to express it to the original Other subsequently or in future application of this task.

Difficulty in Deepening Emotional Experience

Therapist's tone and emotional expression are especially important to further facilitate emotional deepening and communicate to the client that these feelings are welcome and can be held here. When a client is moving towards sadness, a gentle, warm, and caring tone can help to move them to better connect. Likewise, the therapist will attune to any anger emerging, and their tone will have a different volume and intensity to reflect that back to the client. Being highly attuned is crucial for this client group. People with anorexia can vary widely in their emotional expression and therapists should adjust expectations. They may have a flat tone or facial expression that can obscure emotion felt or use restricted language even for emotion that is evidently present. For clients with sensory differences such as those experienced by many neurodivergent people, the amount of sensory information being processed at any one time, alongside other interoceptive differences, can make it a difficult and slow process for clients to 'home in' on the experience and expression of a felt emotional sense. The stance of emotion coach is essential.

Blocks to the Process

In any task, we are listening for disconnection from genuine feeling that may indicate the client has moved from Little Self or Healthy Adult into Critic or coping modes. Common in this task is for a client to surrender to helplessness and hopelessness because the Other is no longer in their life or will never change, or for them to move to the avoidance of a Detached Protector, especially when completed for the first time (and there are likely to be several repetitions with the same Other for resolution to occur). Reflection can be made and empathy given to how stuck this keeps the client or of the fear that runs alongside something held so deeply that perhaps gave them a sense of safety or hope ("If I can just get her to see me and love me, then I will be ok.").

The experience of compassion is seen as a developing process and cannot be forced; it must be genuinely held. A particularly strong block in this stage of the task is the Inner Critic, that tells the client they are undeserving of compassion or care. This block should be acknowledged and explored. It may be enough at this

Table 8.2 Stages in the Unfinished Business Task

Stage	Chair	Description	Useful Therapist Prompts
Stage 1. Identify the Marker & Initiate the Task – *Can We Try Something?*	Self chair	Client expresses lingering unresolved negative feelings towards a significant other (expressing blame, complaint, or hurt about somebody else).	
Stage 2. Express Feelings towards the Other – *Tell Them How You Feel*	Self chair	• Picture the other. • Express feelings (this will likely start at secondary emotion blaming/complaining or compliance). • Listen for client speaking from a coping mode or critic.	• What happens inside when you 'see' her there? • Can you tell her, when I see you there I feel …?
Stage 3. Enact the Other (if Appropriate) – *How Does the Attachment Other Respond to These Feelings?*	Other chair	• Speak and convey the message the client got from the other. • Look for implicit meaning. • Look for implicit (other) emotion.	• What was the message given?
Stage 4. React to the Other and Deepen to Little Self and Core Pain – *Can You Tell Him/Her What Hurts the Most?*	Self chair	• Initial emotional reaction to the other. • Deepen and differentiate emotion to access core pain of Little Self. • Listen for secondary emotions and coping modes blocking the process.	• Can you tell them? When you talk to me like that I feel … • What hurt the most about this?
Stage 5. Express the NEED – *Can You Tell Him/Her What the Little You Needed?*	Self chair	• Client expresses initial NEED. • NEED is elaborated. • Express what was missed or is resented as a result of the need being unmet. • Deepen emotion (to Little Self primary adaptive emotion e.g. grief/sadness and assertive anger).	• Can you (Little Self) tell her what you need?

(Continued)

Table 8.2 (Continued)

Stage	Chair	Description	Useful Therapist Prompts
Stage 6. The Other Responds to the NEED – *Can the Need Be Heard?*	Other chair	Highlight any softening into compassion or rejecting of the needs.	• How do you respond to this? Can you see her pain? How do you feel about her as she tells you this?"
Stage 7. Emergence of the Healthy Adult – *Connection with Healthy Adult Feelings and Action*	Self chair	• Let in self-compassion or setting boundaries. • Support the emergence and 'felt sense' of the Healthy Adult. • Allow and process and adaptive grief.	• What happens inside when you hear that response?
Debrief		(a) Client reflects. (b) Therapist deeply validates any shifts/ non-shifts and praises work done. (c) Make links back to the formulation. (d) Decide on appropriate action (e.g. homework).	

stage in therapy just to note it and direct the client back to the Self, or the Inner Critic chair work from Phase 3 may need further repetitions.

Unable to 'Own' Needs

It is important to note that for some clients the very idea that they can and should have their own needs will be new and difficult to comprehend; it may sit uncomfortably, especially in the context of core shame. This can be common to people with very strong Compliant Surrenderers who have spent their whole lives meeting needs of others at the expense of their own, with those just challenging previously held unhelpful beliefs about emotion, or neurodivergent people pushed to conform to neurotypical standards and crush conflicting (sensory, emotional, social) needs. The therapeutic stance of limited reparenting and empathic responding are crucial here in reflecting that these needs are valid and deserve to be heard and expressed.

Task: Float Back with Rescripting Revisited

Once the 'Unfinished Business' task has been completed and the client has at least partially accessed the Healthy Adult, this can be a useful time to consider revisiting the 'Float Back'. In fact, these two tasks will be repeated and supplement each other during this phase. The therapist should look for and encourage opportunities for this task in subsequent sessions. The task can be completed in line with the instructions provided earlier in this chapter; however, once at the rescripting stage, the client can consider if their own Healthy Adult can now enter the scene in response to the Little Self's core pain and unmet need. It may be that the client does not feel their Healthy Adult would be able to offer them anything yet, indicating more work to assist the Healthy Adult to emerge is needed. The therapist can also suggest that both they (the therapist) and the client's Healthy Adult enter the image together in the first instance. The therapist can attune, coach and guide the client's Healthy Adult to learn to hear and respond to the needs of the Little Self. Here, 'Float Back with Rescripting' becomes a scaffolded self-compassion exercise and deepens relations between the Healthy Adult and Little Self, further expanding the client's view of themselves as somebody with self-agency and power in their life who can attend to, hold, and heal their own pain.

After Clara had rescripted one memory linked with lonely abandonment and shame in which her therapist took the guiding and reparenting role, she was able to access primary adaptive emotions of her Healthy Adult (primarily assertive anger and compassion) during the 'Unfinished Business' task. In one session, she brought a feeling of core loneliness and sadness triggered by a colleague's comment at work which had left her feeling very misunderstood.

This marker for the 'Float Back' task was identified and the task process followed to access an earlier memory resonating with this feeling. Clara described a memory of having tried extremely hard at school aged nine and winning a bronze award. She was aware that her brothers both always won gold awards, but also (although at the time being unaware of having ADHD) Clara knew things were somehow harder for her. She felt shame that she had not achieved more, yet also pride. In the car on the way home from the ceremony, her mum made a flippant recognition of Clara's award and then immediately went on to her brother's upcoming sports event. Clara felt a sudden feeling of sadness and was desperate for her mum to know how hard she had worked and for her to feel proud. When she voiced this, her Mum told her she "might do better next time". Clara began to cry and she was told to "stop being so dramatic" and "stop crying". This is when Clara began to feel an overwhelming sense of loneliness and abandonment. This was the worst part of the memory for Clara, and her therapist encouraged her to connect with the feelings, making them strong in her body, by attending to the felt sense. Her therapist asked Clara what she needed, and she expressed a need to be heard, understood, to know that what she felt was real and ok and to be comforted. The therapist asked, "What would it be like if Adult Clara came in here? Could you imagine that? How could she meet Clara's need?"

Clara said she felt Adult Clara could come into the image and that this could be helpful. Together she and the therapist gently explored what this could look like. When Clara first completed this rescripting and entered the scene as Adult Clara she simply asked for a lift and sat in the back of the car with Little Clara. She quietly told Little Clara, "I see how sad you are. I'm here. You are not alone" and they held hands for the remainder of the journey [Healthy Adult meeting unmet need to be heard, understood, and comforted; showing Little Self compassion]. Later on in this phase of therapy, Clara had experienced greater resolution through repetition of the 'Unfinished Business' task and wanted to revisit this memory. Now when she flagged down the car and spoke to her mum she was much more assertive. She addressed both Clara's mum and her dad, alerting them to Little Clara's feelings and needs, stating that as the adults in the car they should be caring for Little Clara, listening to her, prizing her and validating what she is feeling, and that Little Clara deserved better [Adult Self Setting Boundaries]. Adult Clara again got into the car with Little Clara giving her an emotional hug and again (but much more vocally) showing her compassion for the remainder of the journey.

Building Self-Compassion

Compassion work in therapy differs from work to soothe exposed vulnerability or regulate emotion in a present moment (for this work see 'Working for Optimal Emotion Regulation', Chapter 7). Rather self-compassion is self–self relational concept linked to overall well-being. It enables people to offer themselves safety, security, and self-acceptance. Self-compassion has been described as comprising three overlapping and interacting domains: self-kindness versus self-judgement (taking a caring and understanding stance with ourselves), feelings of common humanity versus isolation (recognising that all people fail and make mistakes; nobody is perfect), and mindfulness versus over-identification (aware of present moment experience neither ignoring nor ruminating on disliked aspects of oneself or one's life) (Neff, 2003).

This description makes plain why self-compassion is so important to SPEAKS, but also that it can most helpfully be explicitly worked with later in therapy for it to be an authentic and meaningful experience. For example, self-kindness requires a softening of the critical voice. A sense of common humanity requires sufficient self-valuation and self-acceptance of what the self 'deserves' and that this should match what others deserve, including the notion that own needs are valued and valuable. Mindfulness necessitates an ability to connect with internal experiences, including emotional pain, and not get caught up in negative self-narrative (over-identification with the critical voice/demanding parts).

Further to this, whilst the critical voice can be an internalised voice of others, particularly those from developmental relationships, so too can self-compassion. People who receive developmental caregiver support engage in self-support, self-praise, and self-soothing later in life (Mikulincer & Shaver, 2007). Therefore, a true connection with self-compassion, especially where it has previously been absent, may also rely on the internalisation of the therapist's empathic compassionate, caring, soothing, and prizing voice, brought via their reparenting stance and empathic attunement during the therapeutic process.

Consolidation of self-compassion is an important inclusion in SPEAKS. Self-compassion can enable clients to keep the critical and demanding parts of self at bay in the future and encourage them to continue to engage with their emotional experience (removing self-interruptions) and in honouring their own needs, thereby supporting the Healthy Adult and its continued growth beyond therapy. There are several tasks that we see as helpful in developing compassionate self-soothing. Note that these include removing the blocks to self-compassion as discussed above. For example, two-chair work to reduce self-criticism also simultaneously significantly increases self-compassion (Shahar et al., 2012).

We are keeping an eye and ear out for signs of self-compassion throughout therapy. Where we notice it, we look to build on it in the moment, where relevant. For example, if a client is using compassionate language in a session therapists can reflect this back, further encourage this, repeat and expand on what is said. They can explore it even further by placing that part of them in another chair and hearing more from that side, encouraging the client to fully connect with that part of themselves using 'Chair Work for Self-compassion'. Building a felt and internalised compassionate voice is an aspect of building and consolidating the Healthy Adult once it has begun to emerge.

Task: Chair Work for Self-compassion

Chair work tasks for self-compassion have been described across several therapeutic modalities, including Compassion Focused Therapy, ST, and EFT (Elliott et al., 2021; Sharbanee et al., 2019; Thrift & Irons, 2020). Simply put, the two-chair task for compassion usually involves putting the Healthy Adult and Little Self in dialogical contact in two chairs so that compassion can be expressed to the core pain and the Self. The purpose is to enhance client's internal validation and care such that they transform their sense of self (e.g., from unworthy or unlovable to worthy and lovable) and offer a counter voice/narrative to the Critic. The task can also go some way to meet unmet attachment needs for connection and care, significantly reducing feelings of being alone and isolated from the world (Reidar Stiegler et al., 2023).

This task can be especially useful here in Phase 4, once the emotion transformation process has been started and a felt sense of the Healthy Adult has been established. Since the task integrates core pain and access to self-supporting, self-soothing, and self-accepting internal resources, this self-compassion task can be particularly valuable when integrated into another task, such as 'Unfinished Business'. See detailed guidelines following and Table 8.3 for summary.

Detailed Guidelines for Chair Work for Self-compassion

Stage 1. Identify the Marker and Initiate the Task – *Can We Try Something?*

The marker for 'Chair Work for Self-compassion' is the client expressing core pain and anguish from the Little Self. Ideally, the client will have at least partially connected with the Healthy Adult in previous work and adaptive emotions been accessed. In such a case, the task can involve a dialogue between the Healthy Adult and the Little Self. This is optimal as it encourages a greater strengthening and positioning of the Healthy Adult and its ability to offer self-compassion. It also builds acceptance of the Little Self and a stronger relationship between these parts, facilitating the reintegrated self.

If this combination is initially too difficult for the client to connect with, other dyads can be proposed, with the Compassionate Other taking the form of: 'Close Friend' (a very close friend the client knows well) or 'Idealised Parental Figure' (parent or other important/significant other relationship, e.g. grandma). The ideal compassionate other would be one who holds the qualities of those in a 'limited reparenting' stance (Thrift & Irons, 2020).

The Little Self can also take a different form if not highly activated at the start of the task. This can be helpful where it feels too 'close' or painful to imagine themselves being offered compassion, or if there is a particularly strong Critic blocking compassion directed towards the Little Self. In this case the client imagines a different scared/lonely/hurt child in the other chair and speaks to them. It can be a child they personally know (someone who is currently a child or somebody imagined as when they were a child) or a 'universal' child. This can be a useful way into the task when self-compassion is still new. Often starting here can still result in the client naturally switching to their own Little Self around Stage 3, so it can be worth checking again during the task who they see or who they are connecting with in the Little Self chair.

As part of initiating the task, the therapist and client must agree on who the adult or child will be. The task does not work well if it becomes too far removed from the client's experience, i.e. if neither adult nor child relates to a part of them. Over repeated completions, the task can be gradually altered (changing the 'selves' in the chairs) to enable the client to 'own' more of the compassion offered to self.

Stage 2. Express Feelings as the Little Self – *How Do You Feel?*

In the Little Self chair, the client connects to and expresses the current pain, anguish and unmet need they are experiencing (or that of the imagined child who is currently having similar experiences to them).

Stage 3. Respond as Compassionate Healthy Adult – *What Do You Want Little You to Know?*

The therapist asks the client to switch chairs and enact the Compassionate Healthy Adult (or Compassionate Healthy Other). Initially the therapist gauges the strength and type of feeling that the Healthy Adult (or Compassionate Other) has for the Little Self ("How do you feel as you see her there?"). This gives an indication of any blocks to offering compassion and further work that might be needed before this task can be more usefully completed. The client who says, "She's so annoying" or "I can't listen to her" is clearly responding from a Critic mode and not compassion; this highlights a different task is more appropriate such as self-soothing for immediate pain or working with the Inner Critic (see Chapter 7).

If the client feels neutrally or at all warmly towards the client, the therapist gently encourages expression of compassion, empathy, validation, and comfort towards the Little Self and their pain. Even those clients who want to respond with compassion can be hesitant here, especially when doing this task for the first time and if never having found these words before.

- "What would you say to her? What is it that you want her to know right now?"
- "Can you tell her, I hear your pain and how it is for you right now?"

Stage 4. Little Self Reacts to Initial Compassion – *Are You Able to Hear This Compassion and Take It In?*

Once initial compassionate messages have been offered, the client changes chairs to the Little Self. The therapist summarises the messages given, emphasising compassion using their own tone and (non-verbal) expression, then explores client's experiences.

- "What's it like to hear this compassion? Can you feel it?"

Some clients will be unable to connect to the compassion expressed and here the therapist attends to and explores these blocks.

- "What stops you?"
- "What would it mean or be like if you could feel it?"
- "What more or what else do you need to hear to be able to connect to or believe the compassion?"

As therapist you are deeply pulling on your empathic and reparenting stance; prizing and empathising with the client's emotional experience, including any inability to accept the soothing and compassion at this time.

Stage 5. Healthy Adult Offers Further Compassion and Addresses Blocks – *What Are Your Specific Compassionate Messages?*

The therapist now asks the client to again occupy the Healthy Adult (or Compassionate Other) chair and respond to the Little Self and to any blocks to letting in the compassion.

The Healthy Adult can explicitly respond to blocks ("Clara, I know that you used to squash your feelings down and the critical part told you that you couldn't cope with your feelings, but we know now that you can be with them and it will be ok."). More specific messages can reflect new meanings in relation to unmet need ("I know that you used to think you didn't deserve any compassion, but we know now that those looking after you should have listened. They were trying their best but should have heard how hard things were for you too. It wasn't ok that your feelings were ignored.").

The client can be encouraged to offer a new core message to the client about themselves and their pain.

- "If you could tell her anything what would it be?"
- "What is it, the bottom line/main thing you want her know now?"

Stage 6. Little Self Expresses Feelings Again – *How Do You Feel Now?*

The client then moves again to the Self chair and the therapist explores what it is like to hear this response to any blocks and the deeper, more explicit and personal expression of compassion and new meanings. The therapist encourages client to turn their attention inwards in response to these expressions of compassion and listens to any shift in emotion, encouraging the client to attend to and symbolise these, particularly in relation to relief, contentment, peace, or wholeness.

Debrief

Once the task is finished, reflecting on the resolution or where the task has reached before the session ends is an important part of the process.

(a) **Client reflects.** Client tells therapist what they notice from the task trying to tease out any meaning made. What do they take away? Ask the client to put into a first person 'I' statement.
(b) **Therapist deeply validates any shifts/non-shifts, praises work done, and prizes emotion shared.**
(c) **Make links back to the formulation.** Clearly connect what has emerged to the mode map and highlight where the new experiences indicate change has occurred or might be needed as a focus of future work.
(d) **Decide on any appropriate action, ideas of different experiences or actions that might be tried between sessions**. Try to keep this collaborative and client directed. Potential homework might be to elaborate what is touched upon in this task using a letter writing task whereby the client writes their Little Self a letter from the compassionate perspective of their Adult Self (note this can also be used as an alternative to this chair task).

Table 8.3 Stages in the Chair Work for Self-Compassion Task

Stage	Chair	Description	Useful Therapist Prompts
Stage 1. Identify the Marker & Initiate the Task – *Can We Try Something?*	Self chair	Client expresses core pain or anguish.	
Stage 2. Little Self Expresses Feelings – *How Do You Feel?*	Self chair	• Connect to Little Self. • Little Self elaborates and deepen core pain. • Little Self expresses unmet needs.	
Stage 3. Respond as Compassionate Healthy Adult – *What Do You Want Little You to Know?*	Compassion (Other) chair	• Identify an appropriate compassionate other, ideally the client's HA. • Respond with initial empathy, validation and compassion to pain of Little Self.	• How do you feel as you see her there? • What is it that you want her to know right now?
Stage 4. Little Self Reacts to the initial Compassion – *Are You Able To Hear This and Take It In?*	Self chair	• Support client to listen to and take in compassion. • Listen for and encourage expression of blocks. • Listen for shifts in felt experience in response to the compassion.	• How does it feel to hear this? • Can you take this message in/believe in it?
Stage 5. Healthy Adult Offers Further Compassion and Addresses Blocks – *What Are Your Specific Compassionate Messages?*	Compassion (Other) chair	• Healthy Adult responds to the Little Self and addresses blocks to letting compassion in. • Further empathy, validation and compassion to pain and unmet need. • Encourage HA to directly express to Little Self and connect to previous learnings if applicable (e.g. what was asserted in the 'Empty Chair' task).	• What is the main thing/ bottom line you want her to know?

(Continued)

Table 8.3 (Continued)

Stage	Chair	Description	*Useful Therapist Prompts*
Stage 6. Little Self Expresses Feelings Again – *How Do You Feel Now?*	Self chair	• Help client to receive compassion and healing of unmet need. • Listen for and deepen shifts in felt sense, including relief, contentment, peace, wholeness.	• Look inside, what happens when you hear this?
Debrief	Self chair	(a) Client reflects. (b) Therapist deeply validates any shifts/ non-shifts and praises work done. (c) Make links back to the formulation. (d) Decide on appropriate action (e.g. homework).	

Moving from Phase 4 (Resolving Core Pain) to Phase 5 (the 'Real Me')

Phase 4 is moving towards Phase 5 when primary adaptive emotion has been accessed and the Healthy Adult who demonstrates assertive/protective anger and self-compassion, and has been able to begin to grieve losses, has begun to consistently emerge. This part may still be tentative, but there is a notable shift in the client's self-organisation that is the foundation for the 'Real Me'.

References

Arntz, A. (2012). Imagery rescripting as a therapeutic technique: Review of clinical trials, basic studies, and research agenda. *Journal of Experimental Psychopathology, 3*(2), 189–208.

Elliott, R., & Greenberg, L. (2021). *Emotion-focused counselling in action.* Sage.

Elliott, R., Watson, J. C., Goldman, R. N., & Greenberg, L. S. (2004). *Learning emotion-focused therapy: The process-experiential approach to change.* American Psychological Association.

Elliott, R., Watson, J. C., Timulak, L., & Sharbanee, J. (2021). Research on humanistic-experiential psychotherapies: Updated review. In M. Barkham, W. Lutz & L.G. Castonguay (Eds.), *Bergin and Garfield's handbook of psychotherapy and behavior change* (pp. 421–467). John Wiley & Sons.

Flanagan, C., Atkinson, T., & Young, J. (2020). An introduction to Schema Therapy: Origins, overview, research status and future directions. In G. Heath & H. Startup (Eds.), *Creative methods in Schema Therapy* (pp. 1–16), Routledge.

Greenberg, L. S. (2010). Emotion-focused therapy: A clinical synthesis. *Focus, 8*(1), 32–42.

Greenberg, L. S., & Malcolm, W. (2002). Resolving unfinished business: Relating process to outcome. *Journal of Consulting and Clinical Psychology, 70*(2), 406–416.

Greenberg, L. S., & Pascual-Leone, A. (2024). Changing emotion with emotion. In A.C. Samson, D. Sander & U. Kramer (Eds.), *Change in Emotion and Mental Health* (pp. 325–344), Elsevier.

Keogh, D., & Timulak, L. (2023). "It's wrong to relax, you have to be on the go, go, go, all the time": Emotional transformation in a case of emotion-focused therapy for generalised anxiety disorder. *Counselling and Psychotherapy Research, 23*(4), 1015–1027.

Mikulincer, M., & Shaver, P. R. (2007). *Attachment patterns in adulthood: structure, dynamics, and change.* Guilford Press.

Milton, D., Gurbuz, E., & López, B. (2022). The 'double empathy problem': Ten years on. *Autism, 26*(8), 1901–1903.

Neff, K. (2003). Self-compassion: An alternative conceptualization of a healthy attitude toward oneself. *Self and Identity, 2*(2), 85–101.

Nimbley, E., Gillespie-Smith, K., Duffy, F., Maloney, E., Ballantyne, C., & Sharpe, H. (2023). "It's not about wanting to be thin or look small, it's about the way it feels": An IPA analysis of social and sensory differences in autistic and non-autistic individuals with anorexia and their parents. *Journal of Eating Disorders, 11*(1), 89.

Pascual-Leone, A. (2018). How clients "change emotion with emotion": A programme of research on emotional processing. *Psychotherapy Research, 28*(2), 165–182.

Perls, F., Hefferline, R. E., & Goodman, P. (1966). Gestalt Therapy: Excitement and growth in the human personality. *Philosophy and Phenomenological Research, 26*(4). 597–598.

Reidar Stiegler, J., Uleberg Vildalen, V., Heggem, T., Båfjord Ismaili, S., & Schanche, E. (2023). The effect of the two-chair dialogue intervention on self-compassion-adding an emotional evocative component to a basic Rogerian condition. *Counselling and Psychotherapy Research, 23*(2), 349–358.

Sharbanee, J. M., Goldman, R. N., & Greenberg, L. S. (2019). Task analyses of emotional change. In L. S. Greenberg & R. N. Goldman (Eds.), *Clinical handbook of emotion-focused therapy* (pp. 217–242). American Psychological Association.

Shahar, B., Carlin, E. R., Engle, D. E., Hegde, J., Szepsenwol, O., & Arkowitz, H. (2012). A pilot investigation of emotion-focused two-chair dialogue intervention for self-criticism. *Clinical Psychology & Psychotherapy, 19*(6), 496–507.

Simpson, S., & Arntz, A. (2020). Core principles of imagery. In G. Heath & H. Startup (Eds.), *Creative Methods in Schema Therapy* (pp. 93–107). Routledge.

Thrift, O., & Irons, C. (2020). Developing a compassionate mind to strengthen the Healthy Adult. In G. Heath & H. Startup (Eds.), *Creative Methods in Schema Therapy* (pp. 269–286). Routledge.

Timulak, L. (2015). *Transforming emotional pain in psychotherapy: An emotion-focused approach.* Routledge.

Timulak, L., & Keogh, D. (2022). *Transdiagnostic Emotion-Focused Therapy: A clinical guide for transforming emotional pain.* American Psychological Association.

Phase 5

The 'Real Me'

Chapter 9 describes Phase 5, which involves a consolidation of processes involved in the emergence of the 'Real Me'. In Specialist Psychotherapy with Emotion for Anorexia in Kent and Sussex (SPEAKS), this has concerned a gradual decrease of reliance on coping modes (such as overcontroller modes, avoidant modes, and surrenderer modes), an increase in visibility of, and cooperative correspondence between, the Healthy Adult and Little Self, occurring alongside quietening of the Critic. In this way, interaction in the world can now be informed by adaptive emotional needs, with the Healthy Adult integrated within the reconfigured and reintegrated self, encouraging self-acceptance, validation, and compassion (Oldershaw & Startup, 2020). In this phase, clients are supported to strengthen the new sense of self and to further internalise the attachment relationship with the therapist through a process of *consolidation of the 'Real Me'*, leading to new ways of being in the world. This final phase of SPEAKS addresses the *ending of therapy*, being sensitive to the 'internal working models' of clients, linked to their early attachment relationships and, with this in mind, guiding clients to express and work through losses and grief.

Consolidation of the 'Real Me'

Reclaiming the Self involves the active exploration and rediscovery of one's authentic identity, resulting in creation or reformation of an identity that is independent from anorexia nervosa (AN) and seen as essential to the recovery process (Dawson et al., 2014; Williams et al., 2016). In SPEAKS, this process to 'authentic identity' is the weaving of a reconfigured and reintegrated sense of self (the 'Real Me'), that moves forward with renewed efficacy and agency. This requires shifting perspectives on, and relationships between, some or all aspects of the Self (e.g. the Eating Disorder Part [EDP]), increasing internal harmony and 'wholeness'. This is seen to occur when the Healthy Adult is guided by primary adaptive emotion of the transformed Little Self (i.e. the client experiences and speaks from a resolved state characterised by adaptive emotions). Means of coping can now be drawn on in ways that regulate and 'hold', rather than overwhelm or dominate, the newly integrated Self. Because often in AN, the EDP becomes such a relied upon

DOI: 10.4324/9781003468349-11

source of identity and may well have developed at a time when identity is naturally fluid anyway (such as adolescence), there can be understandable anxiety, hesitation, and gaps in knowing *how to be* once the EDP and coping modes have stepped back and their roles and control have shifted. Notably, those with lived experience explain that reclamation of the self requires a conscious process, involving deliberate examination of who one is – what they want, need and think – outside of AN (Lamoureux & Bottorff, 2005). A crucial step in recovery is thus the process of reclaiming the non-AN-centric self, occurring in tandem with letting go of AN. This is worked with throughout SPEAKS therapy, utilising many of the tools outlined in this guidebook, not least 'emotion coaching'.

This process of rebuilding the sense of self requires therapists to 'stand with' the person in recovering a sense of identity outside the identity of the EDP (Conti et al., 2020). What this means for this phase of SPEAKS is normalising fears and scaffolding clients to try out wanted new ways of being in the world, taking in feedback and evaluating this via their needs-led Healthy Adult. It is important that clients work towards discovering and reclaiming of the self as 'good enough' (Lamoureux & Bottorff, 2005). 'Behavioural Experiments to Test Out New Ways of Being' that are guided by adaptive emotions and associated needs can support this. 'Embodiment of the Healthy Adult' leads to a greater felt sense of the experience of the Healthy Adult. Chair work to facilitate full emotional expression from the newly emerging Healthy Adult towards the now less powerful and dominant EDP can consolidate this repositioning, and also facilitate a process of letting go in the 'Saying Goodbye to the Eating Disorder' task.

The therapist at this stage is more like a coach standing in the wings, being sensitive to 'Schema Chemistry', mindful that abandonment (ending therapy abruptly or prematurely) and enmeshment (disrupting the process of individuation and prolonging dependence) are both traps not to fall into. The stance here is one of nudging and guiding and prizing the client's experiences, allowing space for a deepening of personal agency and empowerment, as well as being ready to step in and 'holding' where there are inevitable bumps along the road. Tasks from earlier phases can still be utilised even in this phase as markers emerge.

Task: Behavioural Experiments to Test Out New Ways of Being

Behavioural experiments are a key feature of this phase to support new ways of being and relating to extend beyond the therapy space and out into the world. In SPEAKS, this is a gradual process that begins as soon as the client is ready to rely less on coping modes and to be guided by their needs-led Healthy Adult. Behavioural experiments are less formally designed as they might be in Cognitive Behavioural Therapy where predictions are quantified via belief ratings (Rouf, 2004); rather, the emphasis is on planning opportunities for practising various meaningful activities in the world with the individual being 'led' by their Healthy Adult. Clients may also spontaneously engage with something new between sessions. In either case, therapist and client come together to review the outcome enabling further learning and integration. The aim is for interaction in the world to be increasingly guided by the needs of the individual and scaffolded by self-compassion, assertion and new processes that support the central positioning of their Healthy Adult in their Self organisation.

Stage 1. Identifying New Ways of Being

This task begins with identifying new ways of being in the world, or in relationships with the Self or others, that align with the Healthy Adult's needs, goals, and values. The therapist listens out for new client expressions of desired changes and opens a collaborative discussion of what this might look like to try doing differently. It can also be that the client reports spontaneous changes which can be celebrated and reflected on using this process. Any changes should authentically come from the client's Healthy Adult using adaptive emotion as a guide. The therapist should spend some time exploring how suggested changes align with the client's goals for life and values, also assessing the extent to which they may instead reflect a coping mode. This is particularly true for neurodivergent people who have a history of 'masking' (intentionally or unintentionally hiding parts of the self to fit in with neurotypical expectations) to ensure they are not setting expectations relating to 'fitting in' with neurotypical society at the expense of themselves.

During this phase of therapy Clara had begun to express curiosity about relationships. She was aware that she had relied upon her Hider mode (Avoidant Protector) a great deal which meant that her social world had become small. She also grew in awareness that she had tended to occupy certain roles in relationships (People Pleaser mode) in which she would subjugate her own needs and instead tune in to the needs of others as a way of protecting feelings of shame. This meant she tended to assume the role of the 'listener' in relationships, saying little about herself for fear of being rejected for who she was.

Clara and her therapist decided to try out a behavioural experiment. Clara would choose someone she trusted (her best friend who had stuck by her through her years of illness but also knew Clara pre-AN) and engage with that person via her Healthy Adult rather than via a coping mode. Her therapist and Clara practised how such a conversation might go beforehand, and then Clara decided she felt ready and wanted to try. Clara had begun to keep a record of things that she felt proud of each day and she brought her journal entry recording the outcome to her next therapy session:

Initially I sat quietly and asked a lot of questions which is my usual way and I know now part of my Compliant side keeping intimacy at bay because it's scary. After a little while I got brave and I did the grounding into my Healthy Adult exercise and looked over at my friend. I shared something that was somewhat more vulnerable for me; I told her that I was trying to eat out socially but also that this was scary for me and important to my progress. I asked for her for her help in supporting me. She suggested that we buy something here and now in the coffee shop and eat together. She helped me choose something manageable and agreed to have the same. I felt she understood how important this was for me that she was alongside me, so felt scared but decided to go for it. She was so lovely and kind and seemed to really root for me. My Critic tried to ruin things by saying: "Who do you think you are? You know you'll get huge if you do this." But I held onto my Healthy Adult and I just did it. I don't want food to be so powerful. My friend was lovely throughout. I felt warmth towards her and a new kind of connection.

Stage 2. Behavioural Experiments: The Debrief

It is important to have a debrief following an experiment during the subsequent clinical session. Clara's account described the experience from the perspective of 'part selves', showing she had integrated the SPEAKS understanding of Self with the reflective capacity of an anchored Healthy Adult, such that the client is not just 'in' isolated parts of the Self responding. Rather she is 'looking on' with perspective, compassionately noticing her own responses and using her present emotions to guide the interaction. Her therapist guided deeper exploration:

- "What was it like sharing a little more about your vulnerabilities to your friend?"
- "How did it feel?"
- "What did this opening up do to the quality of connection with your friend?"
- "How did this help you to bravely eat with your friend?"
- "How did the Critic respond? And how did you manage this?"

Clara was able to reflect that despite the pulls from the Critic and the compliant side of her, she was pleased she had shifted her role with her friend and expressed some commitment to build on this further. Clara consolidated these Healthy Adult learnings in an audio flash card where she reminded herself that although there can be a pull from her compliant and avoidant sides when trying out new relational challenges, these forms of deflection from her own needs only compound her sense of isolation and sadness, whereas when she is led by her Healthy Adult part, listening closely to adaptive emotions of her Little Self, then she feels empowered and much more connected relationally. Hearing these simple Healthy Adult messages played back to herself in her own voice steadied her when she faced new challenges ahead that pushed her out of her comfort zone.

Stage 3. Continuing New Ways of Being

It is important that behavioural experiments are not single events in time but are built on and repeated and elaborated over time. Helping clients to think about what this could look like even if they don't feel ready to try everything yet can be useful, holding in mind the desires of the client and also the unmet needs identified during therapy.

Being vulnerable with her friend had enabled Clara to test out relational safety to express her feelings and needs. Where this had been feared in the past, her Healthy Adult could hold that these needs were deserved and was starting to believe that these could be truly met in the world. Clara built on this first interaction by initiating a social night out with her friend. Here she connected with under-expressed parts of herself – such as ability for playfulness, child-like fun and spontaneity – previously feared and squashed by the constraints of the eating disorder (ED).

Additional Considerations, Including for Neurodivergent Clients

Typically, behavioural experiments only work out if the client is sufficiently 'ready' and this is indicated by there being a sufficient Healthy Adult part to lead the way. It is also inevitable that these experiments do not go to plan, but this is all part of trying things out initially within the safety of therapy. The debrief can support clients to meet whatever the challenge brought up for them with compassion and acceptance.

The key for this work is not to get things 'right' but simply to have a go at being led by a different part of the self (the Healthy Adult). For neurodivergent clients, the explicit naming and planning of new ways of being may be particularly helpful in managing fears around uncertainty. Recording outcomes in concrete ways supports their integration. Given potentially literal or concrete ways of thinking for this group, it is important to openly discuss that things may not unfold exactly as expected and that this too is ok. Therapist and client can consider some potential ways of managing this. Trying new planned ways of being led by the Healthy Adult and finding oneself able to manage this, especially when things do not go as anticipated, can be a powerful learning experience in itself and go some way to counter anxiety about uncertainty.

For people who have recently discovered that they are neurodivergent, including those who may have understood this for the first time as part of this therapy or have started to see it framed differently, having a clearer understanding of the neurodivergent and ED processes and delineating these or seeing how they have interacted can be very helpful. It is understandable that neurodivergent people may find it hard to feel they can move away from eating disorders when so many of their behaviours have been understood in the frame of the eating disorder diagnosis as opposed to sensory or other neurological difference, which of course cannot be changed. This can leave a person feeling that the eating disorder is intractable, unwavering and inescapable.

A twist on behavioural experiments can involve reframing the understanding of existing behaviour in the context of neurodiversity rather than the EDP, and for the Healthy Adult to use this information. *Clara came to realise that she had made sense of her need to exercise using ED goals of weight loss. Now she knew her*

ADHD diagnosis and sensory differences, she understood it as a response to and way to quieten ADHD hyperactivity and sometimes as a form of 'stimming'. She experimented with listening to different internal energy signals to learn when to stop in the gym, over her previously relied on external measures, such as calories burned. She noticed that she naturally began to do slightly shorter gym sessions and left feeling calm, content, and energised, not depleted as before.

Similarly, lingering body image concerns and anxieties can sometimes usefully be understood in the frame of sensory differences. Our sense of emotional experience reflects active 'top-down' inference of the causes of internal interoceptive signals. This involves some predictive coding around the context of signals, and it requires a reconciliation of sensory input with the level of precision and thus relevance it can be predicted to have (Seth, 2013), i.e. what does this sensation mean and how much certainty can I assign to this conclusion. For neurodivergent people, interoceptive and proprioceptive differences may result in reduced sensory feedback of the body in space. The application of 'top down' inferences based on an eating disorder belief framework, in the context of weak data, can result in 'confirmation' to the client that they are larger than they actually are or are unsafe in some way. Using experiments, this could be challenged and mitigated with sensations of increased pressure that give more accurate feedback of actual size in space, such as weighted toys/blankets, hot water bottles, reducing cognitive appraisals of sensory input as evidence of 'fatness'. This can also change the meaning of sensory feedback to be used as a tool to soothe and not as data of threat (e.g. body size). This importantly differentiates EDP from an integral and unchangeable aspect of neurodivergent brain functioning that ultimately needs now different ways of relating to. Any exploration of the reframing of behaviours and sensations previously tied to the ED should be sensitively done, explored in collaboration with the client and holding a neuroaffirmative stance.

Task: Saying Goodbye to the Eating Disorder

AN often becomes fused with identity and highly valued; it is inevitable that moving away from this part (which has at times been considered a 'friend') will be painful and may trigger attachment anxieties of loss, sadness, and sometimes despair. In SPEAKS, however, the individual is not invited to 'give up' their eating disorder at any point which would likely be resisted or leave an unmanageable gap and a sense of 'who am I now?' Rather the process of SPEAKS is one of a gradual restructuring of the Self akin to a *handing over* of self-management from predominantly coping modes and Critics to the authentic Healthy Adult in correspondence with the Little Self. This handing over means that new self–self relationships are fostered in tandem with other parts, such as the EDP, being dis-identified with. This may mean that this ending phase of SPEAKS involves mixed emotions. There may be recognition of deep sadness and regret at what has been lost over the years along with renewed optimism and energy for the future. Furthermore, moving on from AN as a part of one's identity is also highly distressing. Qualitative studies highlight how recovery can be seen as analogous to loss, and 'letting go' is a key stage (Conti et al., 2020; Williams et al., 2016). A person with lived experience explains: "It's not that I loved my eating disorder but it had become a part of me and my life, so letting go of something, that was so now engrained was a huge thing … for me it was like losing a child." (Broomfield et al., 2021, p.6). Recognition of this loss and making space to process associated grief is thus essential. Indeed, unresolved grief generally can lead to levels of hopelessness, distress, and an inability to adjust to getting needs met in the world in different ways without the lost object (Sharbanee & Greenberg, 2023).

In SPEAKS, the use of chair tasks with the EDP is an iterative process that evolves and transforms over the course of therapy. Thus, chair tasks with the EDP look different, depending on the phase of therapy the client is in and this will impact the goals of the task or where in the task one is likely progress to. Initially, where clients are very enmeshed with the EDP (e.g. Phase 1 and 2), the goals are simply to begin differentiation from it and to hear it as separate. Clients subsequently connect with the impact of the EDP on their lives, thus appreciating the disempowerment that it brings ultimately helping clients see through the 'façade' which can support behaviour change and an enhanced motivation to consider a Self and a life beyond. Gradually, through continued use of the task and emotional processing, clients engage with and express a counter voice (Phases 2–4). Revisiting now in later stages of SPEAKS, when the Healthy Adult is stronger, can support continued shifts in the experienced power of the EDP.

During Phase 5, this chair task explores a process of 'handing over' from the EDP and shifting perspectives on this part, thereby consolidating the newly reconfigured sense of self (The 'Real Me'). For people with AN who commonly experience a core pain of lonely abandonment and attachment fears, saying goodbye to an EDP experienced as an internalised attachment figure will involve further processing of this core pain, affording another opportunity to transform this emotion. Importantly, at this stage in therapy, the task additionally involves processing the loss of the EDP to support 'letting go'. Contemporary models of grief indicate that there are four tasks in processing a loss: (1) accepting the reality, (2) processing pain of the loss, (3) adjusting to a world without the other, (4) remembering the other while embarking on the rest of one's life (Worden, 2018). Chairwork with the EDP here can support a client through these stages, ultimately facilitating grieving, acceptance of loss, and letting go.

Detailed Guidelines for Saying Goodbye to the ED

Below are more detailed notes on the 'Unfinished Business' task and what may emerge or be required from the therapist in each step. This is adapted from earlier descriptions of two-chair work and unfinished business work, as well as work with grief and loss (e.g. Sharbanee & Greenberg, 2023).

Stage 1. Identify the Marker and Initiate the Task – *Can We Try Something?*

The marker for this task is that the client reflects on ways in which the ED may have previously dominated or talks about ways in which they feel they do not need the ED in their life anymore. It can be useful to begin this task where a client has a reflection and is already speaking from the adaptive emotions of the Healthy Adult or there is some re-emergence of the EDP.

Clara towards the end of therapy touched on a moment where she was talking with her therapist about a longing for adult friendships besides her one best friend.

Stage 2. Express Initial Feelings towards the EDP – *Tell Them How You Feel*

PICTURE THE OTHER

The task requires the client to turn their chair to face another empty chair and imagine or evoke a sense of the EDP in the chair.

EXPRESS CURRENT FEELINGS

As soon as the client seems to have a felt sense of the EDP, we want to guide them to their internal experience and immediate feelings towards the EDP. The client is encouraged to express any regret about what might have been in the past if the ED had not been around and to state what they want from the present. The expression and differentiation of any sadness and resentment is encouraged by the therapist to establish the *reality of the loss.*

- "What might you say to your EDP at this point in your life?"
- "Can you express the emotional impact that relying on this part of you has had over the years. What have you missed? What do you resent?"
- "Can you spell out to the EDP the ways in which you need more than this side can offer?"

Stage 3. Enact the EDP – *How Does the EDP Respond to Feelings?*

The therapist invites the client to sit in the other chair and embody the EDP in response to the client's feelings around what has been lost. At first the EDP may push back and say that it is still needed in the client's life; it is still not convinced that the client can move on without them. If this happens, the EDP is encouraged to be specific about why the client still needs them.

The therapist is listening out for the EDP losing its dominance, acknowledging its limitations, and loosening its grip. Sometimes it responds in a quieter tone and the body posture reflects this, rather like the wind has gone from its sails. Here, the EDP may go on to express compassion towards the client, but also its fears about letting go. Again, the EDP is encouraged to be specific about its fears and to amplify the expression of compassion. This may include apologising for the impact it has had.

Stage 4. React to the EDP and further embody the Healthy Adult – *Are You Ready to Say Goodbye?*

The client switches chairs to respond and is encouraged to express their feelings in response to the EDP and its compassion or its tenacity in insisting the client still needs it. This can include expression of the adaptive sadness of grief as the client *processes pain*. Sometimes, even though the client is leaving the EDP behind, they experience feelings of abandonment by the EDP itself, which can result in reaching back for it. The grief of the future loss of the EDP in saying goodbye, in addition to the past losses as a result of the EDP, is explored here.

The client is further supported in any expression of forgiveness and gratitude for what the EDP did for them in the past. Expressions of hope, joy, and gratitude may well be mixed with grief and anger at loss. This reflects *adjustment to a world without the Other* and *remembering the Other while embarking on the rest of one's life*. Therapists validate all of these feelings, supporting their differentiation and expression.

- "It sounds like you can acknowledge the good intentions of the EDP, but now you are also so aware of its limitations …?"
- "How does it fit to thank this side for trying to help you out in the past? What are you thankful for?"
- "Can you let it know that it is no longer needed? Can you say what you will miss? What doors will open for you? What do you long for and hope for?"
- "What would it be like to say goodbye? Is this something you can try?"

Stages 3 and 4 are repeated in a back and forth as grief, gratitude, and resetting of boundaries are expressed.

Clara: For years you kept me stuck and at home and thinking I was unlovable and unwanted, the more I relied on you, the further away from true human connection I got. You offered me empty promises and false hope, and I feel sad and frustrated that you took so many years from me.

Therapist: Can you tell her what you've missed?

Clara: I've missed real relationships, being authentic. Being myself with other people. Really allowing myself to commit to my partner and have a family. I needed to have that, felt so much sadness when I've *watched everyone else in my life settle down. For a long time I thought I didn't deserve it, but now I know I do, I want to try.*

Clara [speaking as the EDP]:   *I never knew you wanted those things. I thought you only needed me. I was scared that you'd get hurt, that you wouldn't be able to cope with that. I'm still not sure you can.*

Clara: *I didn't think I could cope then either, but I feel I'm ready to try. I will miss you though. You were there for me for so long. I'm actually really scared and sad to say goodbye. ... And it feels like saying goodbye is to waste all that hard work, all the years I pushed myself at the gym and didn't eat. What was the point in all of that if I just walk away now?*

Clara [speaking as the EDP]:   *So don't walk away, stay with me. You know you need me.*

Clara: *... the thing is that I know I don't need you. ... I'm sad, but more scared now of staying with you and missing out on my future than I am to leave you behind, even though it is so hard to say goodbye.*

Therapist: *Can you tell her what you're grateful for?*

Clara: *I am so grateful to you for helping me at a time when I felt out of control and at a loss as to how to be in the world. You felt like all I had. I'll always be so grateful for that, and you know, maybe that time isn't a waste as it got me through; you were there for me when I felt alone. And ... I think I can forgive you for what you took, and just be grateful. I'll never forget you and I want to say thank you. I've learnt a lot about myself because of you ... but I'm ready to go. It's true I am scared for the future, but I am determined that there is more to me.*

Debrief

Invite the client to open their eyes and reorient them to the room. Debrief by asking the client to reflect on how the task felt for them.

(a) **Client reflects.** Client tells therapist what they notice from the task trying to tease out any meaning made. What do they take away? Ask the client to put into a first person 'I' statement.

(b) **Therapist deeply validates any shifts/non-shifts, praises work done, and prizes emotion shared.**

(c) **Make links back to the formulation.** Clearly connect what has emerged to changes in the mode map and what this means for the client.

(d) **Decide on any appropriate action, ideas of different experiences or actions that might be tried between sessions.** Try to keep this collaborative and client directed. This work can be supplemented by a letter writing task to the EDP to say goodbye. The task can also be repeated after this to further deepen and consolidate emotions and meaning.

Additional Considerations, Including for Neurodivergent Clients

Blocks and adaptations for this task overlap with those when using chair work with EDP earlier in therapy. Usually, stuck points here relate to the client's readiness for this type of work. If this is the case, using the earlier stage chair work to promote differentiation and decentering and to increase motivation as the client approaches ending will be more meaningful. Common blocks can be re-emergence of the Critic or coping modes, which the therapist should listen out for, as throughout all tasks, and decide whether work with this part may be needed to loosen its influence.

Task: Healthy Adult Embodiment

Taking a focusing stance can deepen connection with the felt sense of self (Elliott & Greenberg, 2021), leading to further development of a part of the self (Briedis and Startup, 2020), as well as developing a specific element such as compassion (Thrift and Irons, 2020). Whilst the HA is emerging, integrating ways to strengthen and consolidate the expoerince and connection with its felt sense is helpful.

Guidelines for Healthy Adult Embodiment

The marker for this task is a clear connection with the Healthy Adult presenting an opportunity for the deepening of its felt sense and presence, by focusing on and exploring related adaptive emotions, action tendencies, and physiological experience. This is perhaps most likely to emerge at the end of another task in which the Healthy Adult has begun to emerge.

The client is invited to sit in a chair and gently close their eyes (or fix on a spot). If necessary they bring to mind a time when they felt in deep connection with their Healthy Adult, using an episodic memory to support their experience if needed. They play out this scene in their mind's eye, in the first person to focus in on that sense of the presence of their empowered Healthy Adult. Therapists support this with exploratory questions.

> *Really try to gather a felt sense of your Healthy Adult. Where in your body do you locate connection with this side of you? How does this feel? Where do you feel this in your body? Can you make this feeling as big as possible?*
>
> *What body posture goes with close alignment to your Healthy Adult? Can you try this now?*
>
> *What images come to mind?*
>
> *What energy or impulses are associated with this side of you?*
>
> *What do you believe about yourself when your Healthy Adult is in the driving seat? Try to say this, "I am ..."*

Really try to focus in on the body sense of your Healthy Adult, try to lean in and deepen your bodily and felt sense of this side of you, try to breathe it in from head to toe and allow this side of you to occupy your full being. Now just be with your embodied Healthy Adult for a few moments.
Only when you are ready open your eyes and return to the present moment bringing your embodied Healthy Adult with you.

Debrief

Once the task is finished, reflect on the process.

(a) **Client reflects.** Client tells therapist what they notice from the task trying to tease out any meaning made. What was this like for them? What do they take away?
(b) **Therapist deeply validates any shifts/non-shifts, praises work done and prizes emotion shared.**
(c) **Make links back to the formulation.**
(d) **Decide on any appropriate action, ideas of different experiences or actions that might be tried between sessions**. Try to keep this collaborative and client directed. Here the invitation can be for them to try out this embodied Healthy Adult mediation daily. The aim is to help them build new connections and new 'ways in' to this side of themselves.

Additional Considerations, Including for Neurodivergent Clients

Some clients may struggle to get a felt sense of this side of themselves and this is ok. The idea is to build this side using as many senses as possible and those most amenable to your client. You may have learnt that your client connects with an emotion via a particular entry point, such as favouring action tendency or physiological experience, and the embodiment can lean into and strongly elaborate these aspects. For some clients choosing a transitional object to represent this side can be meaningful, for others drawing or painting their embodied Healthy Adult can deepen the connection. For autistic people, making the connection back to the original object that was chosen for the Healthy Adult can be useful (e.g. "How might an empowered lion feel?", "Where would they feel that?", "What would their stance be?"), as can using imagery associated with their passionate special interest or any strong connection with nature.

Carrying this work through into life outside therapy can involve further exploration of where they feel their Healthy Adult is strongest in the world or can most easily come to the fore and exploring ways to connect with the Healthy Adult in that environment/relationship more frequently.

Ending of Therapy

A key feature of Phase 5 is managing the relational aspects of ending whilst holding in mind clients' early life attachment history. Ending where clients have dared to attach may reignite a host of fears linked with abandonment and rejection, especially where this has been a core pain for the client. Neurodivergent clients in particular will need reassurance that their therapist is not going to suddenly disappear, and the ending of therapy should be well planned and be expected (Bowers & Widdowson, 2023), avoiding coinciding with other significant life events as much as is possible (Loomes & Bryant-Waugh, 2021).

It is important for SPEAKS therapists to have awareness of their own attachment histories. Clients will not feel able to express and process the pain of separation unless their therapist has worked through their own histories sufficiently to be a 'container' (Delvey Jr, 1985). As therapy comes to an end, what clients need from the therapy space will change; with much more time needed for the processing of grief and loss as well as space to consider how their new identity, new ways of coping and parts of self can take them forwards (Pettersen et al., 2013). These important transitions can only be worked through in therapy if therapists are themselves open to the mixed emotions that can arise at this time, on both sides. There needs to be space to acknowledge regret at what has not been possible to achieve during therapy or clinical change that has been partial (Pattersen et al., 2013). The aim here is for the individual and therapist to meet wherever they are during this phase with curiosity, celebration, reflection, and compassion. This can be supported by the process of reflecting on the parts of self, intrapersonal relationships, and change during the remapping task. A concrete summary to return to is especially beneficial for autistic people with AN (Loomes & Bryant-Waugh, 2021).

During this latter phase of SPEAKS, old ways of coping may resurface as the pain of ending is felt. It is important to pre-empt this and for reactions to the impending ending to be gradually and fully explored. Sessions are usually tapered towards the end to lengthen the time period of this piece of work. It is important that you are working within your client's 'Zone of Proximal Development', which by this point in therapy should enable ways of self-to-self responding previously unavailable to them. One way in which these dynamic processes can be expressed is via the use of the *ending letters*. This is a relational task encouraged from the position of the Healthy Adult and both parties write and (ideally) read their letters aloud to each other to deepen the emotional integration and to share the mixed emotions of sadness and regret alongside hope and renewed excitement.

Reflecting on the pain associated with loss and also the hope that comes with greater independence is encouraged and is a critical feature of this phase. 'Reparenting' is an important relational aspect of SPEAKS and as therapy progresses, the stance is for the client to 'take over' the reparenting in their self-to-self relationship, i.e. for their Healthy Adult to be able to meet the needs and feelings of their Little Self with compassion, attunement, and containment. The expression of this handover can be achieved in the giving of a *Transitional Object* to help clients to 'hold on to' the internalised therapeutic relationship when meeting in person comes to a close.

Client and therapist meet less often, gradually tapering the frequency of sessions to prepare for and process the end of therapy, and deal with any set-backs or emergent situations in the client's life. On average SPEAKS lasts around 40 sessions (Oldershaw et al., 2024) and weekly therapy comes to an end within 9 to 12 months. There should be between one and three follow-up sessions over the next three months, as considered necessary for the client (Oldershaw et al., 2024).

Task: Remapping

At the end of therapy, clients are invited to revisit their parts of self and the relationships between them. This affords a reflection on what has stayed the same and what has changed. Here presents an opportunity to celebrate together and prize changes. It can also alert to work that still needs to be done or things to keep an eye on after therapy. All of the stages in remapping are written and/or pictured and given to the client, for them to use for reflection once therapy comes to a close.

Detailed Guidelines for Remapping

The therapist and client reorientate themselves concerning the parts of self identified at the start of therapy and recognised as therapy progressed. This can involve getting together any objects chosen to represent parts of self.

Stage 1. Explore the Parts of Self and Reflect on Changes

The therapist guides the client to explore their current experience of the different parts of self.

- "Are all of the parts in the same place as they were before?"
- "Have some of them got bigger or smaller?"
- "Have they moved closer to frontstage or further away into backstage?"

The relationships between parts are also explored.

- "Have any relationships between parts changed? For example, have any relationships between parts got weaker?"
- "Have any parts built a stronger or closer relationship with each other? What does this mean for you?"

The therapist explores with the client how they would describe the parts of self now.

- "Are the descriptions of the parts all the same as they were at the beginning? Have any of them changed on the way they behave or interact?"
- "Do you see any of your parts differently now? Or feel differently about them?"
- "What has/hasn't changed in your perception of each part?"

When Clara revisited her remap, she explored and recorded her parts as follows by adding to her descriptions from pre-therapy. Here are some examples of how she explained her parts.

ADULT CLARA

Therapy start: Adult Clara is completely unavailable to me. I just don't know who she is. I wouldn't even include her here.

Now: Adult Clara is here. She knows it is ok to listen out for and take care of her own feelings and needs. She wants to look after Little Clara.

LITTLE CLARA

Therapy start: Little Clara feels lonely and scared. She feels useless and riddled by shame. I don't know what she needs. [this was added to as Clara explored further in therapy and recognised Little Clara's unmet needs for acceptance, connection and care.]

Now: Little Clara doesn't feel so alone and the worthless and shame feelings feel further away. They resurface much less often. Even when they do arise, I respond differently because Adult Clara steps in.

BROADER INNER CRITIC

Therapy start: I can't really identify this as a separate thing, and I hadn't thought about this before. I just know that I am a bad person and useless at everything.

Now: I notice this and have learnt it is the voices of different people from younger life and these weren't true messages for me to hold. When it pops up, I know it is a reminder to connect to Adult Clara and the vulnerable feelings of Little Clara. I spend some time reflecting and understanding what has happened. This helps me break the cycle of automatically jumping into old ways of coping and I can think about what I need.

EDP

Therapy start: The ED is partly a way of coping and partly a criticism. It's something that I feel I had no choice but to follow.

Now: I can see the ED criticises me and also keeps me even more stuck in my ways of coping. I know it is trying to help, but I don't need this now. I have found other ways to meet my needs, like connecting authentically with others. I think if the EDP becomes present again I will know not to take its messages literally and that it is just trying to tell me to something is not right, and I should make time to reflect.

OVERCONTROLLER

Therapy start: I have to know exactly what is happening and be in control otherwise everything will fall apart. I need this part and it is right at the front.
Now: I know that this part is trying to help me, and helping to keep the critic quiet. This part can still be helpful at times, like when I have a deadline for work, as having ADHD can make me feel anxious I'll forget something important. But I know I don't need this help all the time and I can choose when to draw on it instead of it taking over everything and making me anxious and panicky.

Stage 2. Remap

Once the parts of self have been discussed, the client is invited to remap her modes to reflect what has been explored, following a similar format to the initial task outlined in Phase 1.

Clara's remap showed how her balanced part (Healthy Adult) was now more connected and in contact with her emotional Little Self (Figure 9.1). All of her coping modes were still there but much smaller and 'bouncing around' to reflect their flexibility in her life, no longer fixed in place and made rigid by the EDP. While

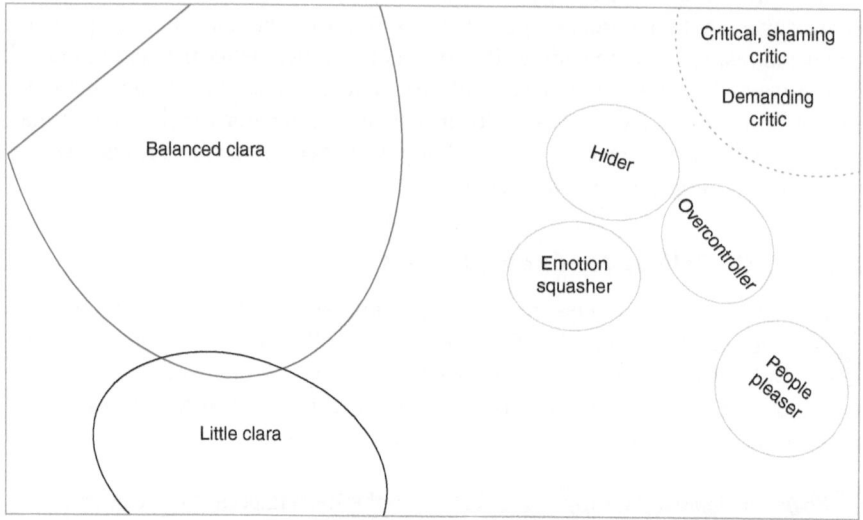

Figure 9.1 Clara's remapped modes

the critical part was of course still present, it was smaller and felt more distant. Clara still used her coping modes to manage it, but they no longer also blocked her Healthy Adult. Clara chose not to put the EDP on her final map, feeling it was not needed.

Stage 3. Finding My Way Back to the Healthy Adult

Once the new experiences of parts of self have been discussed and the remap completed, therapist and client further reflect on how the client will maintain the changes made in the reconfigured self. This includes how to maintain their ability to tune into primary adaptive emotions and use these as helpful guides, as well as continue their meta-awareness of their parts of self and their movement between them. The therapist validates any concerns about moving on and normalises shifts back into old ways of coping, reminding the client that they may still happen and highlighting the importance of finding your way to the Healthy Adult with self-compassion to continue the work, and considering the client's unique tools to do this.

Task: Ending Letters

Ending letters are written from therapist to client and from client to therapist. Ending letters are ideally read aloud (certainly the therapist does this) in one of the final sessions (not the last session). They offer a summary of the therapeutic process and relationship from both perspectives. Letter writing is now a common component of therapeutic approaches. In SPEAKS, although the letter will include a reflection on the formulation and processes of change during the therapy, it may differ slightly from some other approaches because therapists are urged to reflect on their own emotional processes and express their own authentic healthy primary feelings in response to the ending. It is thus not a clinical letter per se, but one of the last ways that they can connect with their client as from one human being to another. This may include self-disclosures such as reflections their sadness that they will no longer see the client and/or their joy at having had this time and to have borne witness to the process and change.

Detailed Guidelines for Ending Letters

Most ending letters tend to be around three or four sides of typed A4. The following is a suggested structure, but this need not be followed exactly, or at all. You should find a way to summarise and express yourself and the work in a way that feels authentic to you. The letter is a continuing expression of the empathy and 'reparenting' stance taken throughout SPEAKS.

- *When you came to therapy* – A reflection on the starting point for the client. This can cover their starting point in relation to you, in relation to their Self, and their hopes for therapy.

- *Your early life* – This is a reflection on the person's background that has shaped their schema and modes and therefore informed the formulation.
- *Formulation and therapy* – A description of how early life experiences have informed the formulation and what the formulation is in terms of different inter-acting modes and intra- and interpersonal patterns. This includes a summary of how this has been approached in therapy, such as tasks, emotions, and changes most significant and poignant. The therapist's emotional reactions to the client's engagement in tasks and what was revealed can be shared here too.
- *Moving forwards* – This is a summary of where the person is on leaving therapy, including a celebration of gains made and acknowledgement of what remains unresolved. The therapist clearly expresses their genuine emotions about the ending, getting in touch with their felt sense about this particular client and their ending, and shares this (as appropriate), rather than what they think 'should' be said. There may be overlaps between clients, but also probably differences.

Debrief

- After both letters had been read, therapist and client reflect on them together. In her letter, Clara was able to express both the multitude of changes she had made during her therapy and her fears and regrets about work left to do. Her therapist used the analogy of therapy as a journey as a way of freeing up Clara from the idea that everything should be 'fixed'; rather, therapy sets in motion new ways of being which, if allowed to flourish via her Healthy Adult, will offer her what she needs going forwards. Clara was able to acknowledge the pain of losing her connection with her therapist, and the therapist could also be open about her sadness and hope for Clara now their meeting in person was coming to a close.
- The physical exchange of letters can function as a valuable transitional object marking the ending of therapy, as well as keeping alive the notion of this as a process now set in motion.

Clara's Ending Letter

Dear Clara,

We have now been working together since September and have come to the end of our sessions. I wanted to take some time to reflect on what I have heard of your story, but also what I have heard of you. I hope I have included everything that feels most significant, but please do let me know if I have missed or misunderstood anything.

When You Came to Therapy

When you first came to therapy, I found you had a lot of questions and seemed to be searching for certainty. This was very understandable with a new therapist who was proposing we work in a different way. I was suggesting that there was not something to 'achieve' each week, but a process of exploration that we would embark on together. It made me aware of how keen you were to make sense of everything that had happened and was happening in quite a concrete way. I could see that dealing with uncertainty was difficult for you, and we talked about how hard it was to try something new, and I was grateful that you were willing to try, but we also considered important factors that could be certain, such as when and where we met and agreeing how we would communicate over physical health management and written summaries you wanted to write and share after each session. It took bravery to take that leap of faith, Clara, and I could see that it was difficult at first (and continued to be uncomfortable at times). However, I felt the trust that developed in our relationship and saw you gradually embrace this way of working.

Your Early Life

Clara you told me about how you were brought up within a very busy household with your two older brothers and parents who were out at work and socialising a lot. You talked about a happy childhood and how good your relationships are with your siblings. Although you knew you were loved and that your parents had the best intentions for you, you described being often made to feel like what you needed or wanted wasn't important and that you were just expected to go along with what everyone else wanted to do. You told me how you often felt lonely and as though you didn't have a voice in your family. There was an emphasis on being fit and healthy, and your brothers were very into sports and exercise, which you could see made your parents proud. You began to set yourself exercise and fitness goals as a way to be seen by and to impress your parents.

Who Am I?

Using two chairs, we began to explore the eating disorder part that told you that you must continue to adhere to the high standards you set during childhood and that you must get everything right just to be accepted. At first you found it hard not to feel defeated by this voice and agreed that it was right. They were such strongly held beliefs, even though you were beginning to see that they did not shape your life in the way you wanted. It told you that it knew what was best and that you had nothing and would fall apart without it. It wanted to block your own self, needs, and emotions. You said that even if you wanted to counter it, you did not feel you had a counter voice yet. We also found there was a part of you that interrupted, blocked, and squashed your emotions. It told you that to talk about emotions was a 'weakness' and not necessary; to show them would make other people reject you and nobody would hear them anyway.

It was in exploring this using two-chair work that you made the direct connection between the critical voice and the voice of your mum. You realised that to reject that (and the EDP) felt like rejecting your mum. You didn't know whether you could do this and weren't ready to let go of wanting to please your mum and the idea that she might still be able to meet your needs.

You have found it hard to reflect on your mum and your relationship with her. There is a side of you that feels it has to prioritise other people's needs and has told you that it is wrong to say anything negative about other people (you called this the 'People Pleaser'). In childhood you were given the message that mum must be protected and looked after, her need must be met at the expense of your own. You started to notice that you walk on eggshells around Mum, and that this happens at the expense of your own needs or emotions. Through addressing your sense of Mum in the chairs, you have been able to express some of your sadness and also frustration. Gradually, over several weeks, through the expression of your feelings and needs, there seemed to be a shift in the way you spoke to your mum in the chair. I heard you express love and compassion towards her as you recognised that she was flawed. This shift enabled you to acknowledge your own valid needs and emotions that were not met in the context of that relationship (to be allowed to be yourself, to rebel and have opinions), and to be able to accept and hold the anger and sadness you have around that. I have seen that you are increasingly able to voice your sadness that you have followed this critical voice for so long and the grief for the life not lived. You asserted yourself in that relationship and were clear, even if it meant her disapproval, this is not the life you want for yourself.

Gradually, over time, Clara, I was excited to see how, in the two chairs, you were able to begin to find the 'counter voice' you didn't think you had. I saw you identify and express your needs to your critical part, the eating disorder part and emotion squasher. You voiced your need for space, to be allowed to try, to be allowed to make mistakes, and to be heard. You began to explore the values and self that you have that are distinct from those impressed on you during childhood and to express these with less guilt and more certainty. You questioned your experience of having ADHD and seeing this as a flaw or deficit, beginning to listen to your associated needs and even feeling excited for the difference it afforded you; something you had previously always hidden. When we used the float back task that last time, you were able to take Balanced Clara into the memory and stand up for Little Clara, showing her care and making sure she was heard and what she wanted was taken into account.

Moving Forward

Clara, at the start of therapy, you expressed a lack of hope that you could ever counter or stand up to the eating disorder part and your Inner Critic. And yet, you have found this part of you that can assert yourself and counter the critical voice that you have known for so long. You have told me how it has started to drive changes in your life, such as having different foods for breakfast, not exercising at the weekend, and having different goals when you do. I loved hearing about your growing and strengthening connections with friends, seeing them even when that involves food. What I have heard you say more and more strongly throughout therapy though is that the pattern you have been stuck in is not a path you want to continue to tread. You want something more and different for yourself in your life;

you have begun to express, explore, and act upon other values that are unique and your own.

Thank you, Clara, for letting me be a part of your therapy. I feel mixed emotions, and I am sad that we won't meet so often now, although I am left with strong feeling of happiness and excitement for you. It has been a joy to see your 'counter voice' grow in strength and enthusiasm and to see your emotional side flourish and guide you. I have so enjoyed getting to know you as the 'Real Clara' emerged more and more during therapy. I wish you all the best as you continue on this path.

Take good care.
Clara's Therapist

Task: Transitional Objects

The exchange of objects can be a valuable way of helping clients to 'hold in mind' the therapy space when meeting in person comes to a close. The key is that these objects are of minimal monetary value but are relationally meaningful in some way and link to an unmet need of the client. Often the transitional object reflects something about the Little Self, the Healthy Adult, or the change process. Even earlier in therapy some clients benefit from carrying around or holding one of their chosen objects linked to a part of self they are working to hold more closely in mind or shifting in their relationship towards. For example, a client struggling to hear emotional needs, may take away the object representing their Little Self to care for and perhaps hold or squeeze gently whenever worries creep in to remember the valid feelings and needs bubbling underneath the eating disorder chatter longing to be heard. At the end of therapy, a therapist can suggest a client keeps the object as a reminder of this most valuable and precious side of who she has become.

During therapy, Clara had described feeling most safe when she could see the sea. She had often visited the seaside with her grandma, and the seafront was somewhere she had retreated to as a child and that still evoked a sense of safety and calm for her in the present. Clara said that as she looked out at the vastness of the sea, she could remind herself that some of the worries that crept in were not so huge, and she could locate herself more peacefully within nature and the universe. As part of the ending, Clara's therapist gave her a small stone from her own local beach as a gesture of recognition and celebration of how hard Clara had worked to reach a place of safety and as a relational gesture to communicate that her therapist held Clara in mind and that relational safety was possible and held between them.

Clara's Therapy Ending

As can be observed throughout this guidebook, Clara's broad changes from therapy reflect those often seen in SPEAKS, spanning cognitive, behavioural, emotional, and relational domains. These shifts drive observable change at the symptomatic (ED) level. Although Clara was a fictional client based within clinical experience, this SPEAKS guidebook hopes to have captured and conveyed some of the depth, emotion, and poignancy of a therapy like SPEAKS and how it can impact upon both client and therapist.

References

Bowers, C., & Widdowson, M. (2023). Transactional analysis psychotherapy with clients who are neurodivergent: Experiences and practice recommendations. *International Journal of Transactional Analysis Research and Practice, 14*(1), 32–54.

Briedis, J., & Startup, H. (2020). Somatic perspective in Schema Therapy: The role of the body in the awareness and transformation of modes and schemas. In G. Heath & H. Startup (Eds.), *Creative methods in schema therapy* (pp. 60–75). Routledge.

Broomfield, C., Rhodes, P., & Touyz, S. (2021). How and why does the disease progress? A qualitative investigation of the transition into long-standing anorexia nervosa. *Journal of Eating Disorders, 9*, 1–10.

Conti, J. E., Joyce, C., Hay, P., & Meade, T. (2020). "Finding my own identity": A qualitative metasynthesis of adult anorexia nervosa treatment experiences. *BMC Psychology, 8*, 1–14.

Dawson, L., Rhodes, P., & Touyz, S. (2014). "Doing the impossible" the process of recovery from chronic anorexia nervosa. *Qualitative Health Research, 24*(4), 494–505.

Delvey Jr, J. (1985). Beyond the blank screen: The patient's search for an emotional container in the therapist. *Psychotherapy: Theory, Research, Practice, Training, 22*(3), 583.

Elliott, R., & Greenberg, L. (2021). *Emotion-focused counselling in action.* Sage Publishing.

Lamoureux, M. M., & Bottorff, J. L. (2005). "Becoming the real me": Recovering from anorexia nervosa. *Health Care for Women International, 26*(2), 170–188.

Loomes, R., & Bryant-Waugh, R. (2021). Widening the reach of family-based interventions for Anorexia Nervosa: Autism-adaptations for children and adolescents. *Journal of Eating Disorders, 9*, 1–11.

Oldershaw, A., Basra, R. S., Lavender, T., & Startup, H. (2024). Specialist psychotherapy with emotion for AN in Kent and Sussex: An intervention development and non-randomised single arm feasibility trial. *European Eating Disorders Review, 32*(2), 215–229.

Oldershaw, A., & Startup, H. (2020). Building the Healthy Adult in eating disorders: A schema mode and Emotion-Focused Therapy approach for anorexia nervosa. In G. Heath & H. Startup (Eds.), *Creative Methods in Schema Therapy* (pp. 287–300). Routledge.

Pettersen, G., Thune-Larsen, K. B., Wynn, R., & Rosenvinge, J. H. (2013). Eating disorders: Challenges in the later phases of the recovery process: A qualitative study of patients' experiences. *Scandinavian Journal of Caring Sciences, 27*(1), 92–98.

Rouf, K., Fennell, M., Westbrook, D., Cooper, M., & Bennett-Levy, J. (2004). Devising effective behavioural experiments. In J Bennett-Levy, G. Butler, M. Fennell, A. Hackmann, M. Mueller & D. Westbrook (Eds.), *Oxford guide to behavioural experiments in cognitive therapy* (pp. 21–58). Oxford University Press.

Seth, A. K. (2013). Interoceptive inference, emotion, and the embodied self. *Trends in Cognitive Sciences, 17*(11), 565–573.

Sharbanee, J. M., & Greenberg, L. S. (2023). Emotion-focused therapy for grief and bereavement. *Person-centered & Experiential Psychotherapies, 22*(1), 1–22.

Thrift, O., & Irons, C. (2020). Developing a compassionate mind to strengthen the Healthy Adult. In G. Heath & H. Startup (Eds.), *Creative Methods in Schema Therapy* (pp. 269–286). Routledge.

Williams, K., King, J., & Fox, J. R. (2016). Sense of self and anorexia nervosa: A grounded theory. *Psychology and Psychotherapy: Theory, Research and Practice, 89*(2), 211–228.

Worden, J. W. (2018). *Grief counseling and grief therapy: A handbook for the mental health practitioner*. Springer.

Index